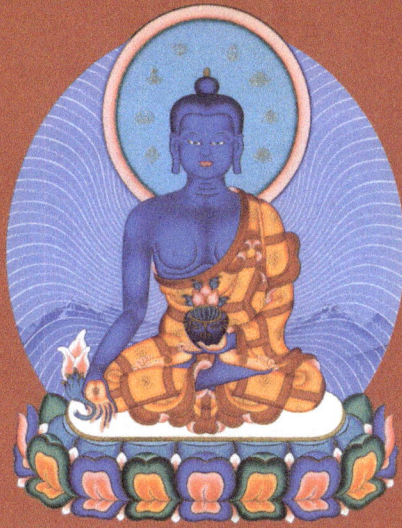

Medicine Buddha

# Dr. Nida Chenagtsang
and Dr Tam Nguyen

# The Tibetan Art
# of Dream Analysis

A journey through space and time...

**SORIG PRESS**

2013

First English Edition 2013
Publisher Sorig Press Limited UK
ISBN 978-1-909738-05-8

Edited by Evelyn Quek

Cover concept and design: Leo Jamorabo

# Contents

*bLa* Energy
Path of *bLa*
*rLung* and Dreams
Emotional Imbalance
Knots
Warnings

## PART 2 – DREAM ANALYSIS TECHNIQUES

## PART 3 – MEANING OF DREAMS

# Foreword

From centuries of practice, Tibetan Buddhism retains great wisdom and knowledge on philosophy, psychology, and the study of thoughts. Naturally, dreams have always been an important part, and are mentioned repeatedly, from Buddha's teaching of *sutras* through to the Vajrayana tantric spiritual text. In the *sutra* the emphasis is more an interpretation of dream symbols. In *tantra* there are very deep levels of the study of dreams, such as dream practice or dream yoga.

In Tibetan medicine, dream study is also a specialised form for diagnosis and prognosis long practised by Tibetan doctors. It is therefore, my fervent wish that this book will provide a deeper understanding of how dreams can heal not just medically but also spiritually.

I thank all my masters, spiritual and medical who have guided me on my own path of learning about dreams. I also thank all my dream students who have supported me and especially everyone who has helped to make the English version of this book a reality, particularly my assistant Dr. Tam Nguyen in transcribing my dream teachings and in her research on the subject, Evelyn Quek for the time spent in editing a complex book, Jean Pierre Kim Chiaverio for conceptualising the cover and Sorig Press for bringing out the book.

Most of all, to my readers, I wish good health and sweet dreams.

DR. NIDA CHENAGTSANG

# Preface

I have always been fascinated by dreams and the clarity of certain ones, one particularly vivid dream floating some forty years in my memory until that dreamt event recently came to pass. As described in this book, dreams of this nature are *prophetic*, foretelling events yet to be. In hindsight, understanding the importance of what was to happen would have prepared me for what was to come.

Through *The Tibetan Art of Dream Analysis* the work of Dr. Nida Chenagtsang, and much of the special knowledge of the ancient Tibetan dream masters originating way back to early shamanic Bon beginnings, is now available to anyone wanting to know more about what takes place during sleep.

We first met in 2008, at the very onset of his teachings and travels in the Far East. Today, centres of the International Academy for Traditional Tibetan Medicine (IATTM) are firmly established worldwide, many books on Traditional Tibetan Medicine written by him, and research initiated.

However, like all good Ngakpas hailing from a secular tradition, it is clear that he sees his work not just from the perspective of a medical practionner but also from a profoundly spiritual one.

It is in this context that *The Tibetan Art of Dream Analysis* has been written, the gift of an open door to ancient practices hitherto passed from teacher to student only by oral transmission and rigorous study.

I never fail to be amazed by his ceaseless energy and special brand of earthy humour, which I suppose is necessary to provide a balanced perspective when one is constantly travelling through various countries and experiencing the intermingling of cultures while attempting to teach and maintain the integrity of a long lineage.

While the book's version in Spanish and Italian is available, the English edition by Sorig Press has not been too late to follow. As editor of the English version, I have taken the liberty to ensure that, despite some of the book's deeply esoteric and spiritual aspects, the main book reads well enough to appeal to any reader interested in studying the rich connection between nightly dreams and their daily lives.

*The Tibetan Art of Dream Analysis* has much to offer everyone. The curious will find Tibetan ideas of dreams based on an interplay between a person's typology, the seasons, environment and the state of mind, highly interesting. Those who are practical will welcome the list of dream symbols and case studies offered, while the more spiritually inclined can follow the detailed approaches in the book leading towards dream yoga's ultimate goal of enlightenment.

It has indeed been my deep enjoyment to play a part in bringing out the English edition of such a rewarding book.

EVELYN QUEK
*Editor*

# A Historical Perspective

Tibetan culture has various ways to explain dreams. It analyses them from a spiritual, medical, or a layman's perspective. But the original source is always the dream itself.

Tibetan medicine, with its 4,000 years of history and sharing a common root with indigenous Bön tradition, is one of the oldest known forms of medical practices. Dream interpretation first appeared in a Tibetan text, the *Yeje Monpei Milam* (ཡེ་རྗེ་སྨོན་པའི་རྨི་ལམ་) with origins dating from an earlier Bön period.

Subsequently, Buddhist theories of dream analysis developed with the spread of Buddhism throughout Tibet by the Tantric master Padmasambhava, also known as *Guru Rinpoche*. The first Tibetan medical texts to talk about dreams were the *Bum Shi* (འབུམ་བཞི), which mentioned the meaning of dream symbols and the various categories they fall into. From the end of the seventh to the beginning of the eighth century, there were two main sources of dream knowledge: one, the medical tradition, refers to the famous Tibetan medical text *Gyud Shi,* (རྒྱུད་བཞི) from the Four Medical Tantras which looked at dreams from a medical perspective. The other, the spiritual tradition referred to in the Vajrayana texts, which contains the Yuthok Nyingthig, (གཡུ་ཐོག་སྙིང་ཐིག), written later in the eighth century, spoke extensively about traditional Tibetan medicine and the practice of dream yoga.

Slowly, various masters or doctors appeared, creating different systems of dream analysis. Two of the most famous Tibetan medicine texts, *Mepo Shallung* (མེས་པོའི་ཞལ་ལུང་) from the fifteenth century, and *Vaidurya Ngonpo,* (བཻཌཱུརྱ་སྔོན་པོ) from the sixteenth century, provided very detailed explanations of dreams. During the 16th century the famous Tibetan doctor, *Desi Sangye Gyamtso*, one of the main disciples of the fifth Dalai-Lama, commissioned a set of *thangkas* to be painted on the study of dreams in the style of his lineage. At that time Tibetan artists painted several aspects of dreams, including its various symbols, and how these would manifest during sleep.

Over time, Tibetan doctors created different systems of dream study. One particular group of Tibetan Masters, called *gTertons,* (གཏེར་སྟོན།) also possessed unique ability to locate *Termas* (གཏེར་མ།) or hidden teachings within dreams, leading to an additional secret practice within dream work itself.

Tibetan doctors use dreams to analyse diseases or illnesses, showing how physical problems are linked to a patient's mental state. But the absence of widespread knowledge of dream analysis made both its study and practice difficult. During the 19th and the 20th Century, great Masters, who were also Tibetan doctors, such as Ju Mipham Namgyal Tso and Tagla Norbu, compiled their knowledge on dreams into a medically coherent system, thereby enabling the systematic study and practice of dreams to this day. Today, Tibetan medicine and its study of dreams offer a long, unbroken lineage of transmitted knowledge.

# Part One

# About Dreams

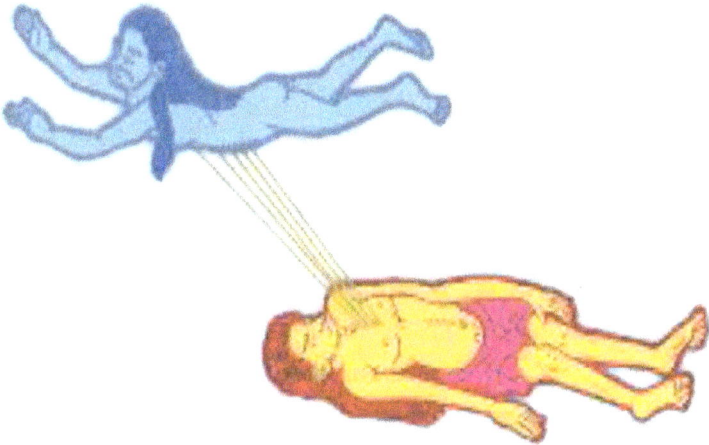

# Sowa Rigpa
## The Tibetan Art of Dream Analysis

Sowa Rigpa (*gso ba rig pa*) refers to the healing knowledge of ancient Tibet. Its meanings are twofold, the first refers to 'healing knowledge' or 'healing science' and the relationship between cause and effect; the second as 'nourishment of awareness' - absolute balance - a perfect state beyond cause and effect possible only through a profound understanding of spiritual traditions.

Many of the principles and concepts in Tibetan culture and its ancient medical system have their origins based on the study of nature, trees, plants and the behaviour of wild animals. This knowledge in turn, provides a context for the delicate balance of perfect health, the types of energies affecting it and how a person may live healthily.

## The 99 'Trees of Knowledge'
Traditional Tibetan Medicine (TTM) is a naturalistic system based on observing nature, and consequently uses symbols such as trees. A complete study of TTM includes the 99 'trees of knowledge'. This is an ancient form of study in which the tree not only represents a person's state of health but also serves as a 'mind map' of all the aspects of Tibetan medicine and its teachings.

Thus the 99 trees of Tibetan medicine are studied sequentially. Previously, 12 years were required to complete a full study of TTM to become sufficiently proficient in its practice. But now, university study in India and Tibet only takes five to six years, with theory taking precedence over practice.

## A Balanced State of Health

Tibetan medicine uses trees as a metaphor to describe an ideal state of health, the first tree with its twin trunks showing both balanced and unbalanced states of health. The first trunk represents a healthy person, in which body, energy and mind are in perfect equilibrium. But if a person's energy becomes unbalanced, then the body and mind follows suit leading to illness. Hence, a balanced state is not just a healthy body, but also refers to the presence of sufficient vital energy and a clear, stable and happy mind.

It is important to note that in Tibetan cosmology, vital energy means a primordial power, the source of all life, also present in the body. This energy arises from the five elements: space, wind, fire, water and earth. At times these elements are considered to be five, and at other times four, as the element of space is the form holding within itself the other four elements. Without space, the other four would not exist. The quality of space is the void giving rise to all phenomena. *Wind* represents movement, growth and development; *Fire* is speed and heat, leading to maturation; *Water*, the character of flow and cohesion, while *Earth* symbolises consistency and stability.

These four elements further distil into three qualities, or energies. The first, *Wind*, comes from the wind element; the second, *Bile*, derives from the fire element; while the third, *Phlegm*, arises from water and earth elements. These three energies further subdivide into two major characteristics of hot (bile) and cold (wind & phlegm) conditions of the human body. Known also as humours or inner energies, they have the following aspects that bring about different functions:

**Wind (rLung རླུང་):** arises from elements of space and wind.
Relates to movement and activity.
Regulates thought and speech.
Controls the nervous system, breathing and excretion.
Covers areas relating to the wind element e.g. head, neck, shoulders, chest, heart, upper abdomen, elbows, large intestine, pelvic bone, wrists, lower abdomen, hips, knees and ankles.

**Bile (mKhris pa མཁྲིས་པ་):** arises from fire.
Relates to heat.
Regulates body temperature.
Covers bodily functions, e.g. digestion, absorption of nutrition, catabolic function, hunger and thirst, courage, motivation and visions.

**Phlegm (Bad kan བད་ཀན་):** arises from earth and water.
Has cold nature.
Covers bodily functions e.g. cohesion, fluid, structural binding of the body, bodily fluids, anabolic functions, sleep, patience and tolerance.

## Tree of Health and Disease (Imbalance)

In analysing different energies and how they are balanced, the first trunk of the first tree shows a healthy human body while the second describes the causes and the types of imbalance. TTM states that all diseases result from incorrect behaviours which in turn create negative karmic conditions. Good karma brings perfect balance or health and bad karma generates imbalance or disease. In TTM negative causes are twofold:

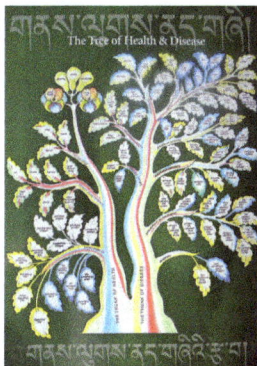

- Primary causes arising from negative, destructive, emotional states such as anger, aggression, lust, unhealthy attachment (desire) and ignorance.
- Secondary causes which derive from persistent and repetitive factors such as wrong nutrition and lifestyle, time factors, (seasonal changes) and external provocations.

Food and lifestyle easily form the main secondary causes of illness. Consider deaths related to cardiovascular diseases. The primary causes tend to be nutrition and lifestyle factors, and awareness of these two aspects can lead to a person being more attentive to getting enough sleep, eating correctly and adopting a better lifestyle. Based on the Buddhist philosophy of "liberation lies in one's own hand." TTM has the same approach that health lies in our own hands.

Time as a secondary cause relates to rhythms and fluctuations of the environment, light, climate and its resulting effects on people. The combined elements in each season affect bodily energies, dietary customs and behaviour of people.

The other secondary cause is provocation. Traditionally, provocation means invisible spirits sending negative energies which influence people and make them sick. The main idea of provocation is that these invisible beings exist and influence the human world. This concept points to the relationship of man with his natural environment. For example when man destroys nature, we set in motion a series of negative events such as the pollution of air and water, a basic cause of many of our current health problems. Regarding spirits, Tibetan medicine believes that as nature is their realm, we should respect their existence and strive to cultivate a harmonious relationship with these unseen forces.

## Tree of Diagnosis

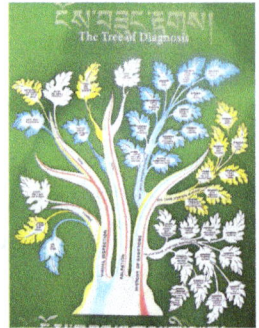

The second tree is the tree of diagnosis and has three trunks:

1. **Inspection – observation**. A patient's behaviour and appearance are examined thoroughly and the first diagnosis made of his urine (e.g. colour, steam, bubbles, smell, sediments, oiliness, and so on).

2. **Palpations – touch diagnosis**. The different pulses of a patient are palpated to assess his particular humour type and health imbalance. Tibetan doctors are trained in a special art of Tibetan pulse reading called *rTsapra* ( རྩ་པྲ་) and in chanting special mantras for a week or a month to increase pulse reading power. This method is not mentioned in the *rGyud-bZhi* but only in the *Yuthok Nyingthig*, being considered a secret practice and known to only a select few.

3. **Anamnesis – case history**. Equally important are questions asked of a patient's lifestyle; for example, diet, sensations, emotional and physical states.

## Tree of Treatment

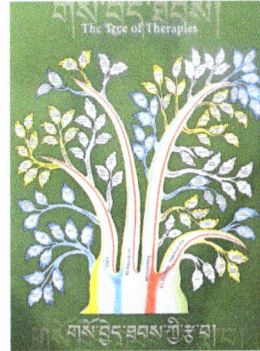

The Tree of Therapies

The third tree of treatment has five trunks of treatments:

1. **Therapeutic Diet** - considered the best form of treatment.
2. **Important Lifestyle Changes** to daily routine, sleep, likes and dislikes, creating considerable impact on a person's health.
3. **Medication** or the use of herbs, minerals and small animal-based substances in Tibetan pharmacology.
4. **Application** of **External Therapies** divided into the use of primary therapies (3rd trunk) such as *Ku Nye* massage, acupuncture, moxibustion and cupping; and secondary uses of herbal baths, blood-letting, compresses, stick therapy and Mongolian Moxibustion.
5. *Mantra Healing*, the fifth trunk according to the *gterma* tradition, is considered to be a treatment in its own right when combined with any of the four treatment modalities described above, and enhances their healing effects. When used with diet, mantras can empower or detoxify contaminated foods. Around the home, mantras may be used to create a more comfortable living space, to improve communication and make work more productive. Written mantras are also worn as amulets for protection against accidents, injury, or to ward off spirit attacks. Used with herbal medicine, mantras can amplify their effects.

During the manufacture of traditional Tibetan medicines, reciting healing mantras releases sound energy into these complex combinations of herbs and minerals. So mantras are often used in combination treatments with external therapies such as *Ku Nye* (*bsKu mNye* (བསྐུ་མཉེ།)) involving massage, acupuncture, moxibustion, cupping, heated stones or herbal compresses. In summary, TTM is both preventive and curative.

## Preventive
Prevention of illness through the correct lifestyle and diet is fundamental to TTM. Most modern chronic diseases like diabetes and heart ailments arise from a mixture of unbalanced mental attitude, poor lifestyle and diet.

## Curative
Once imbalance arises, overt diseases manifest. It then becomes necessary to recreate balance by working on underlying causes and effects, such as diet and lifestyle, before using herbal treatments and external therapies.

# Why Sleep is Important

## Good Sleep is Beneficial

Sleep, a key biological need, is as important as food. As we are not able to survive without food and drink, neither can we live without sleep. One of best ways of resting the mind is to have proper sleep. Good sleep promotes the following qualities of physical and mental health:

. Calm and clear mind
. Mental balance
. Strong energy
. Healthy body
. Body fitness
. Good immune system
. Well-toned organs

In the Four Tantras sleep is mentioned as a key need in a person's life. The text says:

*'Sleep deprivation in the night leads to an increase of harmful characteristics in our body which is why we need a good night's sleep. If one has not slept the previous night, skip breakfast the next morning and try to make up for at least half the period of deprived sleep. Sleep deprivation for those with weak constitutions lead to a person feeling intoxicated, depressed, or exhausted from strenuous activities or even feeling fearful. It may also lead to loss of physical strength and cause instant provocation of rLung disorders in early summer when days are hot and nights are short. To regain sleep balance, taking a nap during the daytime would only increase the oily and heavy characteristics in the body. So sleeping during daytime would aggravate a person's Bad kan qualities and lead to swelling, dullness, headache, lethargy and sus-*

*ceptibility to infection. However, fasting, induced vomiting and having sex can help overcome the effects of excess sleep. The opposite is true for those suffering from insomnia where drinking warm milk, curd, chang or meat broth, applying oil on one's head and putting oil in one's ears help to combat the lack of sleep.*

*In waking state we stay mainly in the consciousness of the intellect. While sleeping this part of consciousness is shut and another opened. In this other consciousness we are capable of having special abilities e.g. terma, learning, discoveries etc. Sleep comes from the chakras and channels in which the eight types of consciousnesses and rLung are circulating. Blockage of this natural circulation causes many problems. Sleeping problems will lead to lack of concentration during the day. It is preferable to sleep on an empty stomach.'*

## Causes of Sleep Disorders

Sleep disorders arise in different ways. At the mental level, sleeping badly can be caused by sadness, grief, stress or being preoccupied. It can also come from eating badly, consuming too light food, drinking too much coffee, tea, or stimulating drinks [e.g. Red Bull], taking too many vitamins, or simply just overeating. An upset or empty stomach can also cause a person to sleep badly.

Sleep disorder can be the result of overwork, physical stress, extreme sports, excessive talking or reading too much. For some, unfamiliar places can disrupt sleeping patterns, as well as the effects of medication. Sleep may also be impaired by changing lunar phases (full, new, and dark moon) or by menopause, a *rLung* disorder.

## Symptoms of Poor Sleep

You are not sleeping well if you find it hard to fall asleep, wake in the middle of the night or too early in the morning. It could be you are already oversleeping, the eventual result being a foggy mind and sleepiness during the day.

## Treating Insomnia

TTM treats insomnia in a many ways:

### Diet

- Drink warm milk with flax seeds or cumin
- Consume broth (meat, bone, chicken etc.) with garlic and onion, vegetable soups with clove and nutmeg and asafetida (*ferula assa foetida*)
- Drink chamomile or fennel tea, warm or sweet wine
- Avoid caffeinated beverages (tea, coffee, etc.)
- Avoid stimulating foods (soft drinks, fruits)
- Avoid medicines or vitamins

### Behaviour

- Relaxation
- Practise breathing exercises or meditation
- If you can't sleep after 20 minutes, do some soft and gentle movements to distract the mind
- Sexual stimulation on self
- Avoid strong movements or exercise
- Avoid stimulating entertainment such as books, television, talking

### Medicine

- Agar 35

- *Dza ti bzhi thang*: nutmeg, clove, ginger, cumin in equal proportions in soups or by teaspoon in powdered form

**External therapies**
- Ear massage with warm oil
- *Hor Me* on the Five Doors of Wind (crown point, centre of the palms and soles)
- *Ku Nye* massage with sesame oil on the head, back of neck, chest, hands and feet
- Moxa on each fingertip and toe tip

**Mantra**
- Recite the mantra *He He La Yo Pak Ta Ya* (ཧེ་ཧེ་ལ་ཡོ་བག་ཏ་ཡ༔), blow on a linseed and eat it
- Recite the mantra *Ri A Hung* (རི་ཨ་ཧུྃ༔)

# Origin of Dreams

## What Is A Dream?

The Tibetan word for dream is *milam (rmi lam* ऋ་ལམ*)*. *Mi* means manifestation, *lam* means path. During the day we release thousands of thoughts, considered by dream practitioners as waves or manifestations. While we are sleeping our consciousness makes its transition allowing these thoughts or waves to become dreams.

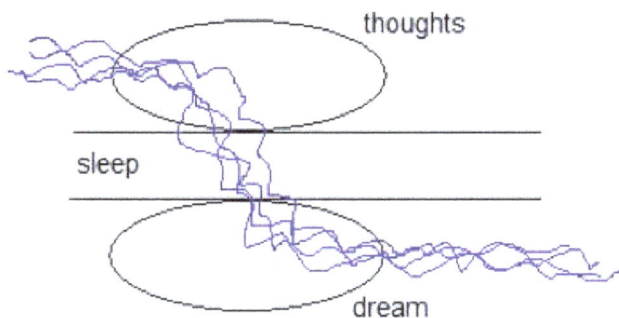

Considered to be reflections of our thoughts, dreams are also much more, being a treasure trove of our mind; our deepest self. Through our fantasies, dreams take us into a magic world where the night spirits communicate with us.

| Reflection of thoughts | Hidden treasure of the mind | Deep understanding of self | Internal journey of the night spirits |
|---|---|---|---|
| Subtle continuous thoughts | New discoveries | Self dimension | Symbols |
| | Deep memories | Self-communication | Fantasy |
| Natural force of mind | Prophetic | Self reflection | Magic |

## Dreaming is Important

### Everybody Dreams

Some people think they don't dream, but actually everybody does even if their dreams can be unclear or easily forgotten. With specially learnt methods dreams become clearer and easier to remember. In rare, well-trained practitioners, the energy moves from the heart chakra into the central channel, where it stays. Usually the energy does not remain here but quickly goes to the left and right channels, where our dream experience begins.

Dreaming is important for all for various reasons, although many people don't attach much importance to their dreams. They therefore would not understand how dreams reflect our physical and mental health, nor its importance to our well-being. Through dreams we understand the links with illness. Both Freud and Jung wrote extensively about dreams, basing their analysis from a perspective of mental illnesses, their research leading to the development in the West of different schools in dream analysis and therapies.

In Tibetan medicine the importance of dreaming lies in five main areas:

1. **Health protection**: Just as our physical immune system protects us from external attacks, dreams act like a mental immune system protecting us from outside mental forces.
2. **Life guidance**: By bringing up past experiences, current situations, or events yet to happen, dreams deepen our understanding of key aspects of our life, for example in relationships or work.
3. **Self-awareness**: All that manifests in dreams comes from self. When learning about dreams we become aware of

these subconscious issues which may not be apparent during waking time. A dream no matter how unusual issues from self, with us ultimately no stranger to it.

4. **Inner guru**: Spiritually, dreams may come from an inner master teaching and allowing us to experience the true nature of all phenomena. For instance, as a dream is a perfect illusion, it may therefore be our only chance to directly experience real illusion without words.

5. **Revealing knowledge**: In dreams we go beyond space and time into other deep realms - an infinite treasure house, full of hidden knowledge. In Tibet a tradition exists, called *therma*, which refers to this hidden treasure, and can be found both in the material and mental dimension. The mental [*mind therma*] is where great practitioners go and find hidden knowledge through their dream or meditation experiences.

## Dreams: Indicators of Health

Tibetan medicine practitioners use dreams to analyse mental problems and assess if a person's mental health is well balanced, and to uncover physical problems. The body is viewed not only physically but also as connected to a person's energies and the five elements of Tibetan cosmology.

Tibetan doctors using their knowledge of the interrelationship between a person's body, energies and the elements are able to use symbols present in dreams to help in curing or preventing health problems.

## Dream Messages

Dreams may contain warnings linked with future events - giving us messages about what is about to happen not just to us but to friends, family or even work colleagues. Being forewarned prepares us to respond more aptly to a particular situation or obtain a better idea of what is important in our present life.

A special purpose of our dreams is to increase our wisdom and understanding. Prophetic dreams and teachings in our sleep state fall under this category

In our daily life, we may encounter situations or problems we are unable to solve, concerning work, study, and people issues. The ability to find solutions through dreaming is a major help in dealing with everyday problems. This is why dreams are very important for our health and mental well-being. In a twenty-four hour cycle we spend an average of seven or eight hours sleeping and dreaming. Some dreams are unpleasant and people naturally dislike bad dreams. However, negativity is part and parcel of living life so it is crucial to try and understand even bad dreams.

To explore how dreams manifest we need to firstly understand the basic components which make up our dreams.

## Components of Dreams

Dreams manifest through our chakras, channels, subtle energies and our consciousness. We have to know what these basic elements of dreams are before starting to interpret them.

| rLung (Wind) | Consciousness | Energy Paths |
|---|---|---|
| Vitalizing energy of life force (biological motion) | Reactions of the consciousness | Channels, Chakras |

## *rLung*

In Tibetan cosmology and medicine all phenomena are based on the Five Elements:

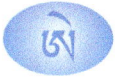 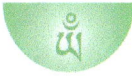 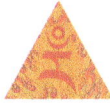  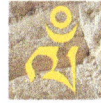

| Space | Wind | Fire | Water | Earth |

They can be further explained simply as:

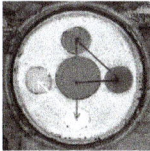

The Five Elements are represented in the Buddhist mandala.

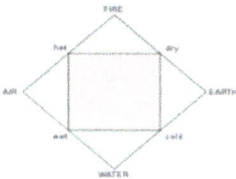

As space is the base of the other elements these can be reduced to the Four Elements as seen in ancient Greek philosophy or "Unani" Greek medicine.

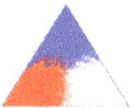

Within space, earth and water (both cooling) combine to become phlegm. The Three Elements or Three Humours system is used in Tibetan Medicine and Ayurveda.

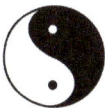

Phlegm and wind combine, becoming hot and cold. (Ref: Traditional Chinese Medicine Yin and Yang).

As shown above, the three humours or energies derive from the five elements, of which *rLung* (wind) is the most important:

- Air or wind energy; *rLung* is the energy of movement sometimes referred to as the dream artist or the actor of our life
- Water and earth energy, phlegm energy; *Bad kan*
- Heat or bile energy; *mKhris pa*

In all Tibetan and ancient East Asian studies, understanding *rLung* is very important especially in dreams as *rLung* plays a significant role. This energy is also known as *prana* (Indian), *chi* (Chinese) and *ki* (Japanese).

*rLung* can be divided into gross and subtle.

| རགས་རླུང་ (rags *rLung*) | ཕྲ་རླུང་ (phra *rLung*) |
|---|---|
| **Gross motion** *las rLung* (karmic or action *rLung*), is more physical. Through the function of interdependence it is the motor for our body. | **Subtle motion** works at a mental level. It is part of our energy pervading space. As all external space is filled with *phra rLung*, there is no difference between space and our consciousness (mind) |

| རྩ་བའི་རླུང་ | ཡན་ལག་རླུང་ |
|---|---|
| (*rTsa ba'i rLung*), | (*yan lag rLung*), |
| 5 root *rLungs*, representing 5 Buddhas | 5 branch *rLungs*, representing 5 Bodhisattvas |

| **Impure aspect** | **Pure aspect** |
|---|---|
| Our normal vision. | ཡེ་ཤེས་རླུང་, *ye shes rLung* (primordial wisdom *rLung*). Is beyond cause and effect. |

*Yan lag rLung* (\*ཡན་ལག་རླུང་) are called branch *rLungs* because they are like small branches *of srog dzin rLung* (སྲོག་འཛིན་རླུང་)— wind that sustains Life. The actual location is the brain and its main function is to activate the sense organs, each of them connected to the internal organs.

## Five Root *rLung* Energies

1. སྲོག་འཛིན་རླུང་ *(srog dzin rLung)*: life-sustaining wind
2. གྱེན་རྒྱུ་རླུང་ *(gyen rgyu rLung)*: ascending wind
3. ཁྱབ་བྱེད་རླུང་ *(kyab byed rLung):* all-pervasive wind
4. མེ་མཉམ་རླུང་ *(me mnyam rLung)*: fire-accompanying wind
5. ཐུར་སེལ་རླུང་ *(thur sel rLung):* descending wind

*Srog dzin rLung*, the life-sustaining wind, is the main *rLung* affecting the other four. Located in the head, it is connected with the emotions, explaining why emotional issues affect our body and why physical problems may cause mental imbalance.

## Five-Branch *rLung* Energies

| *rLung* | Location | Connected organ | Potential | Circulating energy |
|---|---|---|---|---|
| ཀླུ་རླུང་ (klu *rLung*) (naga or snake *rLung*) | eyes | small intestine | vision, self-protection against diseases | actively circulating |
| རུས་སྦལ་རླུང་ (rus sbal *rLung*) (turtle *rLung*) | ear | liver | hearing | strongly circulating |
| རྫངས་པའི་རླུང་ (rzang pa *rLung*) (lizard *rLung*) | nose | lungs | smell | irritates easily |
| ལྷ་སྦྱིན་ཡན་ལག་རླུང་ (lha sbyin *rLung*) (dewa *rLung*) | tongue | heart | spiritual / divine energy, taste | intensely circulating |
| གཞུ་རྒྱལ་རླུང་ (gzhu rgyal *rLung*) (victorious *rLung*) | skin | kidneys | touch | arrow-like |

### Five-Element *rLung* Energies

Another category is element-*rLung*, sometimes considered as part of the branch-*rLung*-system. Depending on the view taken, there could be two or three divisions of *rag rLung* containing as many as 10 or 15 different kinds of winds.

| *rLung* Element |
| --- |
| ཆུ་རླུང་ chu *rLung* (water-wind) |
| རླུང་རླུང་ rLung *rLung* (wind-wind) |
| ས་རླུང་ sa *rLung* (earth-wind) |
| མེ་རླུང་ me *rLung* (fire-wind) |
| ནམ་མཁའི་རླུང་| nam kha'i *rLung* (space-wind) |

## Constant Motion

The first quality of *rLung* concerns movement, which is the real function of this energy. All our physical nature and minds is connected with movement. No movement would mean no development and therefore no function. All functions work through this type of *rLung* energy.

### Blind Horse and Man without Legs

*rLung* begins with our consciousness at the beginning of conception, both starting and developing together. Everyone is aware of how thoughts constantly run through our minds and the perpetual shift of our emotional states. It is this motion of *rLung* which makes our consciousness work. Therefore *rLung* and consciousness work inseparably together creating feelings, emotions, thoughts, concentration, intelligence and memory. Together they result in clarity and light, the mind stimulated into activity by the movement of *rLung*.

This relationship can be expressed as an analogy of a blind horse (*rLung*) and a man without legs (consciousness). A sightless horse cannot see but is still able to stand on its own legs (movement). Similarly, a man unable to walk may still have clarity and see lights (consciousness) but will be unable to find his way (process the information) unless *rLung* is present. In summary, clarity of consciousness would not be able to grow and develop unless movement (*rLung*) is present.

Combining the two, the person 'without legs', can now move with the help of a sightless horse, to proceed in whichever desired direction. The connection between *rLung* and the mind is similar. When they work together, a person will be able to process information efficiently from all the senses. Ignited by *rLung*, consciousness permits emotions and thoughts to take place, creating the capacity of knowing and understanding.

### 78 *rLung* Energies
*rLung* can be divided into ten different categories. A medical text taught by *Shakyamuni Buddha*, a sutra teaching, mentions 78 different *rLung* energies.

### Subtle Breathing
Breath is karmic wind which moves along with our mind. We breathe about 15 times per minute, 900 times per hour, and 21,600 times in 24 hours. Within the 21,600 normal breaths are 674 breaths of *ye shes rLung* which enter the central channel. Of every 32 karmic *rLung*, one becomes *ye shes rLung*. Therefore all wisdom breaths of a whole lifetime total 3 years, 3 months and 3 days (based on 100 years). Counting only the *ye shes rLung*, we would

be perfectly balanced. Unfortunately, most of our time it is connected to the *rag rLung*, giving rise to many opportunities for imbalances. To achieve enlightenment, yogis try to collect all positive possibilities of a single lifetime through concentrating the *ye shes rLung* in these 3 years, 3 months and 3 days.

In subtle anatomy inhaling takes place through the left and right channel. Energetically the breath goes through the channels to all the organs, first to the head, then throat, heart, and finally navel. Later, returning in reverse. However, if the breath is held, the wind stays and enters the central channel. Whereupon the mind stops having dualistic visions and stays very calm, since there is no movement in the central channel. This is the only place where our energy works free from cause and effect, being charged with wisdom wind. There are three phases of *rLung* breathing: *jug* ( འཇུག) inhaling, *gnas* (གནས་) holding and exhaling *bjung* (འབྱུང་).

Generally, quicker breaths age the body faster. With shorter breaths our body and cells work overtime. If we can hold our breathing longer, our cells relax; our bodily movements slow down, becoming calmer and quieter. Some yoga exercises teach slow breathing techniques, all yoga movements emphasizing holding the breath. Being able to hold the breath deeper and longer prolongs the body's life force.

Up to the age of 25, we inhale more; from then till 45 we hold our breaths longer as our energy becomes more balanced and energetically matured. After 45, exhaling becomes predominant, a point where our memory starts to weaken, we lose hair, and so on. Through slow breathing however, we will be able to retard the ageing process.

Subtle breath does not go only from the nose to the lungs and back, but is connected to all channels and chakras. The subtle aspect of our breath has **five rainbow colours** which can only be perceived through meditation. If the complete length of the wind energy is 28 fingers long, when we inhale the length of 13 fingers enters our body, while 15 fingers stay outside. As the colours are distributed differently over this length, different colours occur through inhaling and exhaling. This is called element breathing. Part of our breath is taking something inside and throwing something out. Another part is constantly moving between inside and outside. Extreme sports are considered negative, since the external breath becomes too long, shortening our lifespan.

Through deep breathing and holding, even without yoga, karmic wind transforms into wisdom wind, the best remedy for all diseases, since all disturbances have their source in *rLung* imbalance. For any imbalance, relaxation is always beneficial as calming the mind relaxes the wind which can be alleviated by also using *rLung* therapies such as *ku nye* and *hor me*. Relaxation prevents *Bad kan* and *mKhris pa* disorders, which are driven by *rLung*.

## Breathing Yoga

A special yoga exercise, called *bum ba chen* or vase breathing especially useful for beginners to calm the mind and in preparation for meditation, involves inhaling, holding, and moving the belly. This sends the karmic *rLung* from the lateral channels to the central channel. The method requires five counts each of inhalation, holding and exhalation, a breathing cycle repeated 21 times. By so doing, a special energy field in the navel chakra is built and the breath divided into a superficial, upper breath and a lower, deeper holding one. In the beginning a novice might feel dizzy after a few deep breaths, but if this is done every day for 20 minutes, the body becomes used to it and the capacity to hold develops, from 10, 20 or even 100 breaths. By training in this manner, our body energy is strengthened considerably.

This technique may be combined with visualisation and sound. Inhale with '*Om*', hold with '*A*', and exhale with '*Hung*', this mantra being the natural sound in our breath. For the visualisation exercise *rLung ro selwa*, which means 'eliminating the dead wind', inhale the five element colours through the skin seeing them inside, cleaning your body and energy.

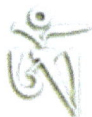 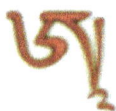 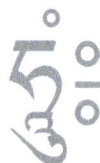

| **Om** | **A** | **Hung** |

## Other Divisions of སྤྲ་རླུང་ phra *rLung*, Gross *rLung*

### *rLung according to gender*

| Energy | Sex | Quality | Channels | Corresponding pulse |
|--------|-----|---------|----------|---------------------|
| *po rLung* | male | short and rough | extremes of success or failure | *rLung* |
| *mo rLung* | female | soft and gentle | positive experiences, stable development, smooth life | *mKhris pa* |
| *ma ning rLung* | neutral | balanced | little experiences & development | *Bad kan* |

### *rLung according to lunar and solar energy*

| *tsa rLung*: hot (horse *rLung*) | *drang rLung*: cold (yak *rLung*) |
|----------------------------------|-----------------------------------|
| quick, sharp, going with solar energy | slow, dull, going with lunar energy |

### rLung according to location

| sTeng rLung: upper | og rLung: lower |
|---|---|
| from navel upwards, influences diseases in the upper body | from the forehead downwards, influences diseases in the lower body |

### rLung of the 9 orifices

| rsog rLung: rLung of life | rTsol rLung: rLung of effort |
|---|---|
| sTeng rLung (upper wind) | og rLung (lower wind, gas) |
| jug rLung (inhaling wind) | jung rLung (exhaling wind) |
| gYon rLung (left wind) | ye rLung (right wind) |

# Consciousness, a *Dzogchen* Tradition

Tibetan medicine looks at consciousness according to *Dzogchen* teachings based on the medical texts written by *Yuthog Yonten Gonpo* (The Younger) a Buddhist Master in the *Dzogchen* lineage.

## The Three Levels Of Consciousness

Consciousness according to *Dzogchen* tradition is divided into three levels, the first being the six senses, considered as the *outer* part; the second level, the subconscious the *intermediate* part; and the third level, root consciousness, the *inner part*.

In all, there are eight types of consciousness expressed as:
. Five Senses Consciousness
. Mind Consciousness
. Emotional Consciousness
. Base (Root) Consciousness

While the subconscious (emotional consciousness) is the dream's leading actor, mind and senses play an important supporting role. These connect the outer five senses and mind with the inner base consciousness. Here, in the subconscious, lies our ignorance, working as we sleep and dream. The five senses and the mind consciousness connect to the material level of existence. Their base form the consciousness of the eyes (sight), nose (smell), tongue (taste), ears (hearing), skin (touch) and mind (analysing). We use these senses to conduct and organise our daily lives. The clarity and purity of the root consciousness is the true nature of our mind. Linking with the other two types of consciousness, it shows an ever present path to pure, clear consciousness.

If **consciousness** can be likened to a tree, the **root consciousness** would be the roots, the **subconscious** the trunk, and the six senses its branches. The three different levels of consciousness are connected by the different layers of emotions, all linked in turn to the subconscious, explaining why we dream. Therefore, our dreams are connected to everyday emotions, though in dreams we look at things objectively compared to seeing them more subjectively in waking state.

**House of Consciousness**
The root consciousness is like a house, and the subconscious a person who walks in, bringing all sorts of emotions, views and opinions collected from outside, the doors of the house being the six senses. Everything a person brings into the house from outside is kept within. In our dreams we look inside the house where we selectively view the objects we have collected. The subconscious is always making a copy of what we think, see, hear, smell, taste, touch including all our impressions of those sensations, which are then stored and naturally reflected in our dreams.

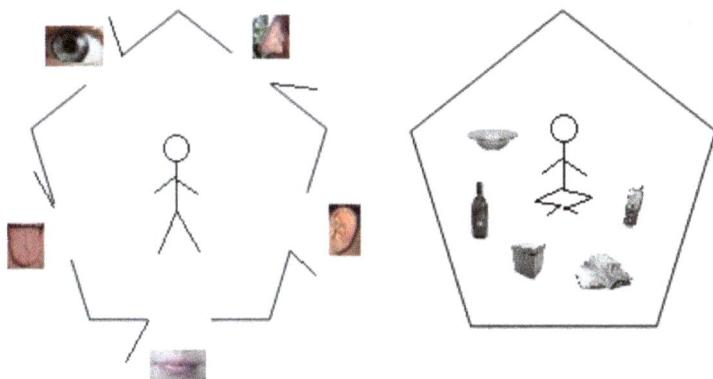

## Brain and Heart

While awake we are fully cognitive or conscious, in sleep state we are non-conscious, functioning within our subconscious mind. While asleep, our subconscious circulates throughout our body. According to Tibetan medicine, just after birth, or when the consciousness is completely awake, two main types of consciousness can be found in the **brain** and **heart** of the new physical body. The **main consciousness**, termed as being 'imprisoned in the brain', is located there where the six sense organs also reside. The special channels of *rLung* or wind energy, link the brain to the heart, these last two connected to the chakras, themselves, an integral part of dreaming. Our wide variety of emotions or feelings is further divided into fifty-four categories.

## Channels

The word ཙ *rTsa* meaning root also refers to: blood vessels (veins and arteries), nervous system, tendons, ligaments, channels, meridians, and so on.. In subtle anatomy, *rTsa* means energetic channels and chakras which have no karmic or dualistic aspects unlike physical parts of the body such as the spine or the aorta.

Channels and chakras can only be seen by developed internal vision. They may appear as forms of very thin, subtle and moving aspects with different shapes and sizes, some reaching body size while others merely half a finger long.

## Channels of Different Sexes

All channels within each person relate to male, female or neutral energy. This is alluded to in old paintings of Shiva, half male, half female. Western medicine itself accepts that women may have lesser male hormones and vice versa, but that male and female hormones are present in both gender.

### Presence of male and female channels

| Channels based on gender | Meaning | Description |
|---|---|---|
| *Pho rTsa* | Male channels | Tight, with many knots. May be used positively but can be dangerous as both extremes are possible. |
| *Mo rTsa* | Female channels | Straight and smooth, without knots. Usually beneficial and less troublesome |
| *Ma ning rTsa* | Neutral channels | Neutral quality without extremes. |

There are many different channels and chakras, but there are primarily the Three Root or Queen Channels, and the Five Chakras.

### *dbU ma* (དབུ་མ།): Central Channel

The ending *-ma* refers to female, like in 'mama'. *U Ma* is the central mother. The size of the central channel is like the thumb. With visualisation it can be reduced or enlarged. Various Tibetan medicine texts may refer to different sizes, mainly a result of the visualising mind.

The central channel has four characteristics which are very similar to the blue colour at the base of a flame:
- thin and transparent
- internally red light, externally blue
- straight
- clear

In our body the central channel is like a black hole in the universe. It has energy to absorb everything into its void including sucking in the karmic wind and making it disappear into emptiness. When this happens, dualistic vision ceases.

There are four instances in which central channel experiences can occur:
- **Orgasm**: All energy enters the central channel after a strong orgasm. If the sexual energy is too strong and you stimulate your nose softly, the sexual energy can transmute. When the energy goes in the central channel our mind becomes non dual. Often we lack awareness of this happening. If not, we would have a split second vision beyond dualism.
- **Sneezing**: Seconds after sneezing produces a feeling similar to that after an orgasm.
- **Deep sleep**: At the moment of sleep, the energy goes to the central channel which is different from western deep sleep phase, when all brain functions are lowered.
- **Moment of death**: At the moment of our last breath, our consciousness experiences non dualism before fading.

These experiences usually last only a few seconds, not long enough for us to recognize them clearly. The central channel is responsible for all spiritual experiences, *rLung*

41

entering the central channel gives rise to different experiences and visions, such as perceiving very strong lights in certain practices, deep blue smoke or clouds. Spiritual experiences show the nature of the energy entering the channel – transforming karmic *rLung* into wisdom *rLung*. *Yuthok* gives precise explanations about this. But in unstable minds, practice of this type can be dangerous and very often visions are mere hallucinations instead of true central channel experiences. When this happens, it is often the sign of a sick *rLung*. The spiritual aspect of realization lies mainly with the central channel. *Saraha*, the famous first Indian Buddhist yogi says, "When our *rLung* and our consciousness enter the central channel, all our common or normal perception completely disappears." He means that at this moment, our mind is no longer dualistic, as we experience realisation.

### ཚོ། & རྐྱང་མ། *Ro ma* & *rKyang ma*: The right and left channel

Starting at the nostrils, both channels wind around the central channel at each chakra, before returning to their respective sides, entering below the navel into the central channel. *Ro Ma* is on the right side, *Chang Ma* on the left.

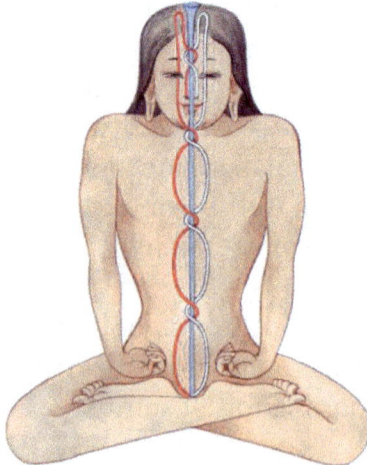

### རྩ་ངན་ *rTsa nGan*: Negative Channels

As there are positive channels *rTsa bZang* (རྩ་བཟང), there are also negative channels *rTsa nGan* (རྩ་ངན་), one type being undesirable channels *mi dod pai rTsa* (མི་འདོད་པའི་རྩ་). Mental aggression and anger grow the negative channels which can increasingly manifest in our body, just as in a beautiful garden bad weeds may proliferate to the point where flowers die. In the same way the negative channels can grow and kill positive ones. Each person creates his or her own bad energy. So while a person may appear physically healthy, internally disturbances could be at work.

If a person full of negative channels is dying, these negative channels, carried as karma within the body, will lead towards a negative direction. Positive channels growing in the body will consequently lead to a positive path. Or negative channels could die allowing positive ones to take over.

Six negative channels called *Obstacles of the Vajra Body* may create obstacles in a person's spiritual practice, too many of these impacting even the body. We could be born with them or grow them through bad karma. But negative channels can be purified through positive karmic actions and the recitation of the *Vajrasattva* mantra.

| Negative channel | Meaning | Effect |
|---|---|---|
| *Nyal ma* | sleeping channel | Sleepiness during meditation. |
| *Shar ma* | paralyzing channel | Pressure or tension during spiritual practice. |
| *Böng ma* | reproductive energy channel | No orgasm or sexual sensation due to excessive negative channels creating difficulties with reproductive energies or becoming pregnant. Obstacles in tantric practice. |

| Negative channel | Meaning | Effect |
|---|---|---|
| *Dong ma* | hole channel | Causes loss of energies and lack of pleasure sensation. |
| *Zing ma* | mess channel | May be compared to too many traffic lines mixed together. Overly present, makes person prone to diseases. Pain and illness increase during spiritual practice. |
| *Chu ma* | deforming channel | Causes deformed or bent babies. Too many present makes spiritual practice difficult with no progress. |

## གདོན་རྩ། *don rTsa*: Demon Channels

Another type of *min dod pai rTsa*, **undesired channels,** are གདོན་རྩ། *don rTsa*, demon or provocation channels. There are five channels through which provocations can enter. All demon channels lead to the ring fingers or toes. Negative activities or thoughts open these channels, through which demons may easily enter. With positive thoughts, even if a demon enters, it leaves again because of boredom.

Demons attack different organs, sending bad energy from their entry points throughout the body. They can also suck energy through the channels.

To diagnose a provocation pulse, urine, symptoms and dreams have to be considered. Wearing rings, especially with precious stones on our ring finger or toe, or tying with a red ribbon or thread, are protective measures which close up the entry points of demon attacks.

| Demon channel | Meaning | Affected organs |
|---|---|---|
| *tsan rTsa* | red spirit channel | lungs |
| *gyal rTsa* | evil king channel | heart |
| *ma mo rTsa* | female spirit channel | liver and kidneys |

| Demon channel | Meaning | Affected organs |
|---|---|---|
| *theurang rTsa* | one-legged spirit channel | stomach |
| *lu rTsa* | naga channel | small intestine |

## A demon story from Shabkar's biography

*One day Shabkar felt a big demon coming to him. It entered through his mouth. Shabkar felt pain everywhere. He did tum mo practice and used fire to burn the demon. The demon then suffered from the heat. He knocked at the belly and said:*
   *"Please let me come out! "*
*Shabkar said:*
   *"You entered through the mouth; you must exit through the arse. "*
*Then he farted and the demon was released.*

*The next day another big spirit came to him.*
*He said:*
   *"I am sorry that one of my spirits disturbed you. He was the head of the demons. You shamed him - you burned and farted him. "*

## Natural spirits on different days

| Weekday | Spirits | Meaning |
|---|---|---|
| Sunday | Tsen | Fire spirit |
| Monday | Za | Planet spirit |
| Tuesday | Gongpo | Jealousy spirit |
| Wednesday | Sadak | Earth spirit |
| Thursday | Songma | Protectors |
| Friday | Mamo | Female spirits |
| Saturday | Jachin | Indira |

## Chakras

If we liken the three channels to the main trunks of a tree, the chakras would appear as knots from the branches. Chakras are central points, where many channels converge to form a sort of wheel, *khor lo* (འཁོར་ལོ།). In all Tibetan studies, religious, traditional or medical, the study and use of the chakras is widely understood. However, the number of chakras may differ; some Tantric schools refer to seven chakras, others four or five. Some schools may even use as many as eighteen chakras, whereas *Dzogchen* teachings sometimes use only two.

### The five root chakras:

- The head chakra

- The throat chakra

- The heart chakra

- The navel chakra

- The sexual chakra

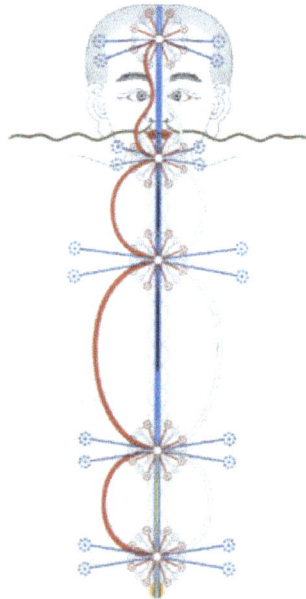

Tibetan medicine uses five chakras. The type of chakra or the numbers of chakras mentioned differ according to the practice or teaching referred to although the basic chakras stay the same. Chakras are always linked and have a special relationship with each other. But whether we refer to one, two, five, six, seven, or even eighteen chakras, the root number in Tibetan medicine is always five. There are other commonly known chakras, such as *the third eye* located between the eyebrows or the *navel chakra* located just below the navel and the *crown chakra* found at the crown of the head. The five basic chakras, combine the smaller chakras in the head with the main one. These basic chakras are important in study of dreams because, while dreaming, subtle energies circulate through them.

| Chakra | Petals | Features |
|---|---|---|
| ཀྱི་བོ་བདེ་ཆེན་འཁོར་ལོ་<br>*spyi bo bde chen 'khor lo*<br>Head chakra<br><br><br><br>*chakra of great pleasure* | 32 | The head chakra energy is very important in Tibetan medicine. At the physical level the head chakra is reflected as the brain, which is called *the ocean of the nerves*. From here they descend to every part of the body. |
| མགྲིན་པ་ལོངས་སྤྱོད་འཁོར་ལོ་<br>*mgrin pa longs spyod 'khor lo*<br>Throat chakra<br><br><br><br>*chakra of enjoyment* | 16 | Has a double face. Called the enjoyment chakra as it enjoys different tastes, connecting to breath, speech and voice power. Energetically very important as it is one of the bases of staying balanced.<br><br>The throat chakra produces dreams being the entrance to the dream world. |

| Chakra | Petals | Features |
|---|---|---|
| ཤྱིང་ག་ཆོས་འཁོར་ལོ་<br>*snying ga chos 'khor lo*<br>Heart chakra<br><br>*chakra of phenomena* | 8 | The eight petals of the heart chakra are connected with the 8 consciousness (5 senses, mind, base consciousness, and, subconsciousness).<br><br>Heart is the base of consciousness. An upset mind disturbs the heart chakra and the physical heart. Emotions may block the heart channels. Syllables, vibrations and different kinds of *rLung* are connected to the heart chakra. |
| ཏེ་བ་སྤྲུལ་བ་འཁོར་ལོ་<br>*let ba sprul ba 'khor lo*<br>Navel chakra<br><br>*chakra of manifestation* | 64 | The navel chakra consists of 12 base petals contained within 64 petals, their inner energetic pathway an exact image of the solar system and the zodiac, a day's inner circuit equal to a calendar year. Called the reincarnation chakra it is also the base of manifestation. Human life (foetus) 'starts' from the navel, our subconsciousness staying in this area capable of generating strong emotions. Avoid cuts, punctures, operations, acupuncture, piercing and tattoos here as they damage the channels. |
| གསང་གནས་བདེ་སྐྱང་འཁོར་ལོ་<br>*gSang gNas bDe sKyang 'khor lo*<br>Sexual chakra<br><br>*chakra that maintains the great pleasure* | 32 | During orgasm consciousness resides in this chakra. Through visualisation, it is able to generate the special heat of tummo.<br><br>Visualise a white energy - the letter *hung*, upside down, on top of the central channel, and at its bottom, 4 fingers below the navel, a red triangle. A thin, red hot flame from the triangle goes up the central channel melting the hung and releasing a drop of white energy downwards.<br><br>The central channel experiences the non-duality of great bliss being generated in the head chakra, melting and spreading down till it reaches the lowest chakra, the maintenance of great bliss. |

## Dakini Points

The first four chakras each have eight different points similar to subtle moxa points, called *Dakini* points. They are located in a circle which contains a picture of a dancing *Dakini*. Each chakra point, itself a *Dakini*, has therefore *Dakini* energy and a syllable related to the point.

*Dakinis* are female deities who have accomplished spiritual realisation. The energies of the channels are considered as female energy, even in men. The reason being the foetus stays in the mother's womb for almost a year and although the sperm comes from the father, most of the energy is derived from the mother. Each point has its own functions. When a chakra is unbalanced it will show in the points. If the points are disturbed by external causes, the chakra can be affected, much like a flower with damaged petals. But the damaged energy of the points can be reactivated through meditation, mantras, yoga exercises or massage.

The 32 *Dakini* points are related to the macrocosm, each point on our body connected to 32 energy points on our planet. Although physically, we must travel to these places to receive their energy; energetically they are already present in us. Therefore problems occurring in nature or worldwide would have an impact on our health.

| Head Chakra | | |
|---|---|---|
| Dakini Point | Location | Effect on |
| རྩ་མི་བྱེད་མ་ *rTsa Mi Byed Ma* inactive Dakini | Fontanel | Teeth, Hair |
| རྩ་ཕྲ་གཟུགས་མ་ *rTsa Phra, gZugs Ma* thin Dakini | Hair part | Hair |
| རྩ་བཟང་མོ་མ་ *rTsa bZang Mo Ma* benevolent Dakini | Right ear hole | Skin |

| Head Chakra | | |
|---|---|---|
| Dakini Point | Location | Effect on |
| ཙ་གྱོན་མ་ rTsa gYon Ma<br>left Dakini | Occiput | Muscles, Left Body Functions |
| ཙ་འདུལ་བྱེད་མ་ rTsa Dul Byed Ma<br>conquering Dakini | Left ear hole | Tendons, Ligaments |
| ཙ་རུས་སྦལ་མ་ rTsa Rus sBal Ma<br>turtle Dakini | Forehead | Bones |
| ཙ་སྲིད་པ་མ་ rTsa sRid Pa Ma<br>existence Dakini | Between eyes | Kidneys, Spleen |
| ཙ་དབང་བསྐུར་མ་ rTsa dBang bsKur Ma<br>empowerment Dakini | End of clavicle | Thighs, Calves |

| Throat Chakra | | |
|---|---|---|
| Dakini point | Location | Effect on |
| ཙ་སྡང་མ་ rTsa sDang Ma<br>angry Dakini | Arm pits | Kidneys, Eyes |
| ཙ་བཤུང་བ་མ་ rTsa bShung Ba Ma<br>shitting Dakini | Nipples | Liver, Gall Bladder |
| ཙ་མ་མོ་མ་ rTsa Ma Mo Ma<br>primordial female Dakini | Navel | Lungs |
| ཙ་མཚན་མོ་མ་ rTsa mTsan Mo Ma<br>night Dakini | Tip of the nose | Small Intestine |
| ཙ་བསིལ་སྟེར་མ་ rTsa bSil sTer Ma<br>cooling Dakini | Palate | Ligaments, Tendons, Periosteum |
| ཙ་གྲོ་བ་མ་ rTsa Gro Ba Ma<br>lucky Dakini | Neck | Abdomen |
| ཙ་ནགས་ཚལ་མ་ rTsa nags Tshal Ma<br>forest Dakini | Chest point 8 | Stool |
| ཙ་མཆུ་མ་ rTsa mChu Ma tear Dakini | Perineum | Clitoris, Testicles |

| Heart Chakra | | |
|---|---|---|
| Dakini point | Location | Effect on |
| ཙ་ཐུང་གཅོད་མ་ rTsa Thung gCod Ma<br>cutting Dakini | Urethra | Mind, Consciousness |

| Heart Chakra | | |
|---|---|---|
| Dakini point | Location | Effect on |
| རྩ་གྱུང་གཅོད་མ་ rTsa mDzes Ma pretty Dakini | Urethra | Mind |
| རྩ་རོ་བཅུད་མ་ rTsa Ro bCud Ma taste-of-food-Dakini | Urethra | Mind |
| རྩ་ཀུན་ཁྱབ་མ་ rTsa Kun Khyab Ma all-pervading Dakini | Urethra | Mind |
| རྩ་གསུམ་སྐོར་མ་ rTsa gSum Skor Ma three-cycle-Dakini | Eyes | Eye consciousness |
| རྩ་འདོད་པ་མ་ rTsa 'Dod Pa Ma desire Dakini | Ears | Ear consciousness |
| རྩ་གཏུམ་མོ་མ་ rTsa gTum Mo Ma wrathful Dakini | Tongue | Tongue consciousness |
| རྩ་བདུད་འདུལ་མ་ rTsa bDud 'Dul Ma demon conquering Dakini | Skin pores | Skin consciousness |

| Navel chakra | | |
|---|---|---|
| Dakini point | Location | Effect on |
| རྩ་མདོག་མཛེས་མ་ rTsa mDog mDzes Ma beautiful-colour-Dakini | Genitals | *Bad Kan* |
| རྩ་ཐུན་མོང་མ་ rTsa Thun Mong Ma general Dakini | Anus | Large intestine |
| རྩ་རྒྱུ་སྐོར་མ་ rTsa rGyu sCor Ma health-giving Dakini | Thymus | Blood |
| རྩ་བྲལ་བ་མ་ rTsa Bral Ba Ma separating Dakini | Calves | Sweat |
| རྩ་མཛའ་བོ་མ་ rTsa mDza Bo Ma *friend Dakini* | Fingers, Toes | Fat, Bone Marrow |
| རྩ་གྲུབ་པ་མ་ rTsa Grub Pa Ma *accomplishing Dakini* | Wrists, Ankles | Tears |
| རྩ་མེ་མ་ rTsa Me Ma fire Dakini | Back of the Hand, Big Toe | Mucus, Saliva |
| རྩ་ཡིད་འོང་མ་ rTsa Yid Ong Ma attractive Dakini | Patella | Mucus, Snot |

# Manifestation and Dream Types

## Dreams in Science

Our sleep is regulated by an inner biological clock. This is a completely natural process comprising of neurological, psychological and hormonal reactions.

Western science states that people have 2 types of sleep: REM (rapid eye movement) and non-REM. According to our brain waves our state of consciousness falls into the following types.

| State | | Brain waves | Features |
|-------|--|-------------|----------|
| awake state | | fastest brain waves | no dreams |
| closed eyes | | medium brain waves | no dreams |
| non-REM | first light sleep state (shortly after falling asleep) | slow brain waves | sleep starts, muscles twitching. While dreaming muscles are paralysed |
| | second sleep state | slow brain waves with irregular waves in between | sleep gets deeper |
| | third sleep state (transition into deep sleep) | slowest brain waves | sleep gets deeper |
| | fourth sleep state (deep sleep) | | older people may not reach this state |
| REM | REM sleep | fastest brain waves | dreams in this phase are much easier to remember |

At night, when we sleep, we go through this cycle five or six times. The longer we sleep, the shorter the fourth sleep state gets and the longer we stay in the light/REM sleep. By morning we may or may not have reached deep sleep state.

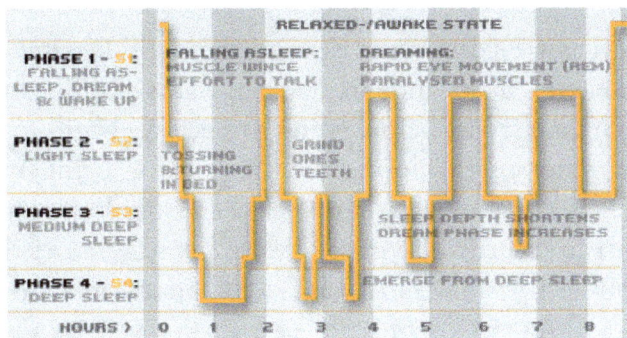

| | RELAXED-/AWAKE STATE | |
|---|---|---|
| **PHASE 1 - S1:** FALLING ASLEEP, DREAM & WAKE UP | FALLING ASLEEP; MUSCLE WINCE EFFORT TO TALK | DREAMING: RAPID EYE MOVEMENT (REM) PARALYSED MUSCLES |
| **PHASE 2 - S2:** LIGHT SLEEP | TOSSING & TURNING IN BED | GRIND ONES TEETH |
| **PHASE 3 - S3:** MEDIUM DEEP SLEEP | | SLEEP DEPTH SHORTENS DREAM PHASE INCREASES |
| **PHASE 4 - S4:** DEEP SLEEP | | EMERGE FROM DEEP SLEEP |
| HOURS ⟩ | 0    1    2    3    4    5    6    7    8 | |

http://timon-royer.com/en/8/refreshing-sleep-everyday/

## Manifestation Pathway

To understand how consciousness comes into being, how *rLung* functions, the channels, position and appearance of the chakras, we have to start with how dreams manifest.

*How do dreams manifest?* Firstly, the subconscious circulates via *rLung* which, in turn, moves through the following four states of consciousness (*gnas skabs bzhi*):

. The conscious, awake state, as we live our daily routine, experiencing pleasure and pain, talking, listening and perceiving life through the senses.
. The deep sleep state, when we are not dreaming.
. The dream state, following the deep sleep.
. The state when we experience orgasm, just before fainting or sneezing.

During any of these four states the *rLung* is also circulating around the chakras. As there are five chakras and four states of consciousness it means that one chakra is always at rest.

Usually our subconscious and our main *rLung* are moving around the navel chakra, where we experience emotions through the six senses.

As soon as we sleep the senses and the mind become calm as the energy floats and circulates upwards via the left and right channels. Just before going to sleep we begin to relax as the mind softens, losing the sharpness of being awake. As the energy moves upwards, closer to the heart chakra, we start to feel the heaviness of sleep because the earth energy builds up in the heart chakra. When the subconscious and *rLung* move closer to the heart chakra we relax further, our mind becoming foggy. From here as energy enters the central channel we fall into deep sleep. When the energy enters the central channel we do not have dreams, feelings or emotions as we are in total, profound relaxation.

## Location of the subconscious during the four different states

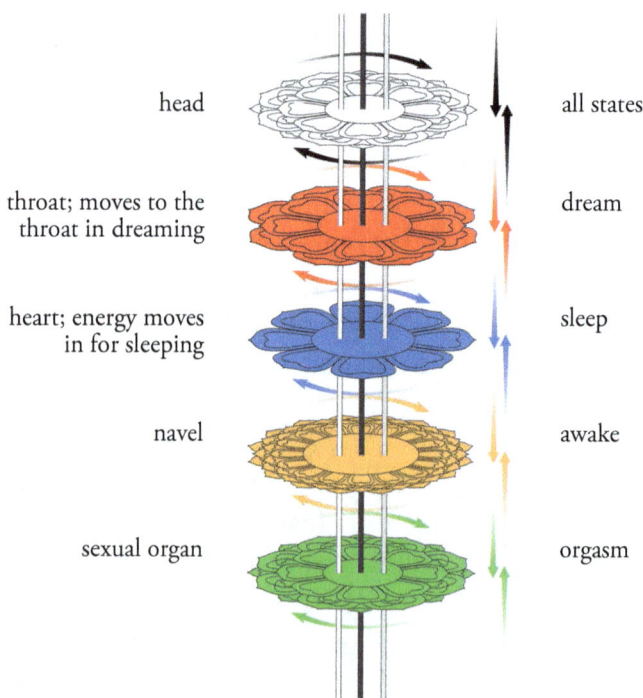

| | |
|---|---|
| head | all states |
| throat; moves to the throat in dreaming | dream |
| heart; energy moves in for sleeping | sleep |
| navel | awake |
| sexual organ | orgasm |

In many tantric teachings such as *Yantra Yoga* the practitioner tries to move *rLung* into the central channel. One outcome of successfully transferring this energy is sustained deep relaxation, a similar feeling to falling into deep sleep state.

In most people the energy emerges from the central channel, travelling up the throat chakra via the left and right channels within the first few minutes of deep sleep. The throat chakra is linked to the head chakra and as the energy and consciousness circulate through this area, we start dreaming.

The head chakra is linked to the sense organs for seeing, hearing, tasting, touching and smelling. As the *rLung* reaches the head chakra we again experience feelings, sensations and visualisations, and although asleep, we are able to see and hear sounds as clearly as if we were awake. The energy continues to move around different parts of the head chakra; if it moves into the stronger part of the chakra we experience sensations such as seeing clear light or very illuminated objects. If the energy moves onto a different point, we hear different sounds or voices of people with a heightened sensation of hearing.

When we start to wake from this dream state the energy slowly circulates downwards from the head chakra to the throat chakra, the heart chakra and on to the navel chakra. In an awakened state the energy no longer enters the central channel, travelling directly from the left and right channels down to the navel chakra. The speed of waking depends on the flow of this energy, as people with more phlegm energy tend to wake more slowly, whereas those with more bile energy would wake faster.

During a 24-hour cycle the energy travels up from the navel chakra to the head chakra and back down to the navel chakra. The chakra at rest during this circulation process is the base or sexual chakra; only awakening when a person experiences an orgasm. When the subconscious and associated energies move to the base chakra, it activates.

If the energy remains in the central channel, even if it is moving up and down, no dreams will appear. Certain high level yogis can practise this way, holding the energy in central channel, their state of mind remaining in clear light and not dreaming. This is called **Clear Light** (*'od gsal*) practice. The mind experiences a profound state of awareness in a deep rest state in an adept practitioner to the point where he or she is able to sustain energy within the central channel.

The ability to access G*ong Ter* (mind g*Terma* ) is connected with the true nature of the mind, the root consciousness.

Thus the subconscious connects the root with the six sense consciousness. Our dream state is due to the workings of the subconscious. When the subconscious enters the root consciousness we may experience clear light and the real power of the mind enters the dream. In that state everything can be understood and the *Gong ter* (*mind gTerma* གོང་གཏེར།) appears.

Our dreams, our mind and consciousness are all linked with the chakras and channels, so clarity of mind and all sensations depend on these as well. The circulation of our energies, time of day, external environment and astrological influences determine the condition or state of our circulating energies. It is important to note that, astrologically, our circulating energies have an energetic connection with the sun and the moon. For instance the sun rises in the morning and shines through the day before night falls, the cycle repeating the next day. Similarly our inner energy goes up with the first light and descends as the day darkens.

## Dream Experience

Dreams are influenced by various factors such as the physical and mental state of the dreamer or the environment, expressed through a variety of dream phenomena. Our perception and actions in the dream state depend on these inner and outer factors. As the connections to these factors are complex it may not be always easy to trace dream experiences back to their original source. But we can explain how common phenomena may manifest through dreams.

### Common factors influencing dreams

| Elements | Energy state | Time | Health state |
|---|---|---|---|
| Environment and element | Typology | Astrological connection | Organs, mental and energetic imbalances |
| Predominant colours | ↓ | ↓ | |
| | rLung dreams | Dreams of beginning, mid and end of night | ↓ |
| | mKhris pa dreams | | |
| | Bad kan dreams | | Dream symbols |

### Perception in Dreams

We have to understand what really happens when we dream as we might not recall anything when we wake.

### Why do we see colours in dreams?

In dream analysis colours are a manifestation of the elements. Each colour is associated with a different object or form and connected to bodily functions. The elements and energies in our bodies consist of different colours, reflecting as such in our dreams. Colours also manifest from channels and chakras and from our imagination. If we repeatedly imagine or visualise a colour we eventually see it in dreams. How well this is done depends on the intensity of the practice. Many *rLung* practices correspond to different *rLung* energies, each expressed in a different colour.

In dreams we may experience all the sensations we feel when awake - hear sounds, speak, eat, taste, touch and smell. These sensations are linked to our elements or energies. Further, the five chakras connected to the five elements are expressed in different colours; for example, the blue heart chakra connects with the element of space. Although each chakra contains all five elements - earth, water, fire, wind and space - one element always predominates. These five elements also form a mandala in all parts of our body with one element in each of the four gates of the four directions, the main element always located in the centre.

As we descend into sleep, energy enters the heart chakra, thereby increasing the earth element which accounts for the experience of heaviness. Colours in dreams generally depend on the condition of the channels in which the subconscious and *rLung* energies are active. Channels which are grey in colour denote a weakened state, such people dreaming mainly in black and white, indicating the presence of weak elements. Through relaxation dreams can become more colourful appearing bright and clear as the dream yoga practice intensifies.

## Time and Dreams

The relationship between time and dreams is explained in Tibetan medicine by their connection to astrology. The kind of dreams we have differ according to the period of dreaming. Dividing dreaming time into three periods (beginning, middle and end), during each period our energies may increase excessively, decrease rapidly or appear disordered, their levels influencing our dreams. The imbalances of the three energies or humours *rLung*, *mKhris pa* and *Bad kan* referred to frequently in dream analysis, give rise to different types of diseases. If balanced, this indicates general good health. The three humours influence dreams. The beginning part of the night is influenced by *Bad kan*, the middle by bile or *mKhris pa*, and the end of the night or early morning by *rLung*.

| Time | Cycle of humours |
| --- | --- |
| 8 pm – 11 pm | phlegm manifestation |
| 11 pm – 12 am | phlegm transition to bile |
| 12 am – 3 am | bile manifestation |
| 3 am – 4 am | bile transition to wind |
| 4 am – 7 am | wind manifestation |
| 7 am – 8 am | wind transition to phlegm |
| 8 am – 11 am | phlegm manifestation |
| 11 am – 12 pm | phlegm transition to bile |
| 12 pm – 3 pm | bile manifestation |
| 3 pm – 4 pm | bile transition to wind |
| 4 pm – 7 pm | wind manifestation |
| 7 pm – 8 pm | wind transition to phlegm |

## Time, a Seasonal Influence on Dreams

| Season | Features |
|--------|----------|
| རྒུན་སྟོད་<br>*dgun stod*<br>early winter | Pores constrict; power of internal heat and equalizing wind increases. Eat the first 3 tastes -sweet, sour and salty, meat soups and oily foods. Apply sesame oil and wear warm clothes. Warm oneself by hot fomentation, fire or sun rays. |
| རྒུན་སྨད་<br>*dgun smad*<br>late winter | In late winter phlegm accumulates in the abdomen. |
| དཔྱིད་ཀ་<br>*dpyid ka*<br>early spring | The digestive heat declines as the sun warms and phlegm rises. Eat the last three tastes - bitter, hot and astringent, old roasted barley, meat of dry land animals, honey, hot boiled water, ginger decoctions, coarse, powered food and liquids. Vigorous walks, rub flour on skin; sit in fragrant, shady groves. Use emetics to cleanse |
| སོས་ཀ་<br>*sos ka*<br>late spring | Stronger sun deprives. Take sweet, light, oily and cool, powered foods. Avoid salty, hot and sour tastes. Bathe in cold water, wear very thin clothes. Cool, fragrant houses, shady trees, moist winds and light southern breezes are beneficial. |
| དབྱར་ག་<br>*dbyar ga*<br>summer | Rain power and cool wind but body is scorched by the sun's rays. Bile accumulates. Take sweet, sour, salty food - and warm powered food and drinks. Wear camphor, khus khus grass scented clothes; sprinkle rooms with cooling fragrances and water and cleanse body with suppositories. |
| སྟོན་ག་<br>*ston ka*<br>autumn | Bile rises. Cool food and astringent medicines. |

## Astrological Influence on Dreams

| Day | Mon | Tues | Wed | Thur | Fri | Sat | Sun |
|-----|-----|------|-----|------|-----|-----|-----|
| **Planets** | Moon | Mars | Mercury | Jupiter | Venus | Saturn | Sun |
| **Dreams** | blue | red | blue | green | white | yellow | red |

## Elemental Combinations Influencing Dreams

| Combination | Effect |
|---|---|
| earth-earth | Auspicious: wish-fulfilling energy fulfils all the wishes of an individual |
| water-water | Auspicious: refined energy strengthens and extends life |
| fire-fire | Auspicious: gives prosperity for gain in wealth and property |
| wind-wind | Auspicious: sublime energy quickly accomplishes wishes |
| earth-water | Auspicious: productive energy brings great happiness in life |
| fire-wind | Auspicious: powerful energy brings good luck |
| earth-wind | Inauspicious: unfavourable energy reduces growth of wealth and property |
| water-wind | Inauspicious: incompatible energy to separate loved ones |
| earth-fire | Inauspicious: burning energy generates suffering |
| fire-water | Inauspicious: death energy leads to loss of life |

## Astrological Animals

| 12 Astrological Animals | Cycle time | Day cycle |
|---|---|---|
| Mouse | 0 - 2 | Midnight |
| Buffalo | 2 - 4 | After Midnight |
| Tiger | 4 - 6 | Early Morning |
| Rabbit | 6 - 8 | Dawn |
| Dragon | 8 - 10 | Sunrise |
| Snake | 10 - 12 | Getting Warm |
| Horse | 12 - 14 | Midday |
| Sheep | 14 - 16 | Afternoon |
| Monkey | 16 - 18 | Late Afternoon |
| Bird | 18 - 20 | Sunset |
| Dog | 20 - 22 | Getting Dark |
| Pig | 22 - 24 | Late Evening/Night |

At times when we dream of animals, these may refer to people and their astrological signs. If we dream of ourselves as an animal and something negative happens to this animal in our dream, it could mean that we received a bad astrological influence. But if the animal appears healthy and strong, then astrologically, the sign is positive. When I was in Tibet someone told my master a dream. This person dreamt of a tiger that was in trouble. My teacher found out that the astrological sign of the person was indeed tiger and told him that the tiger he dreamt was himself. As it turned out, he was experiencing health and work problems caused by unfavourable astrological combinations. Therefore based on a negative animal/week day combination bad dreams can occur as well.

**Animal/Week Day Combinations Affecting Dreams**

| Astrological sign | Positive day | Favourable day | Unfavourable day |
|---|---|---|---|
| mouse | Wednesday | Tuesday | Saturday |
| buffalo | Saturday | Wednesday | Thursday |
| tiger | Thursday | Saturday | Friday |
| rabbit | Thursday | Saturday | Friday |
| dragon | Sunday | Wednesday | Thursday |
| horse | Tuesday | Friday | Wednesday |
| snake | Tuesday | Friday | Wednesday |
| sheep | Friday | Monday | Thursday |
| bird | Friday | Thursday | Tuesday |
| monkey | Friday | Thursday | Tuesday |
| dog | Monday | Wednesday | Thursday |
| pig | Wednesday | Tuesday | Saturday |

During the waxing moon dreams are more peaceful whereas during the waning moon the likelihood of more disturbing or action dreams is greater. Besides dreams, the five astrological elements exert an influence on a person's health as well.

## The Five Basic Astrological Elements

| Element | Wood | Fire | Metal | Water | Earth |
|---|---|---|---|---|---|
| Form | Oval | Triangle | Semi-Circle | Round | Square |
| Colour | Green | Red | White | Blue | Yellow |
| Function | Light | Hot | Sharp | Fluid | Heavy |
| Qualities | Growing | Burning | Hard | Wet | Stable |
| Direction | East | South | West | North | Intermediate |
| Seasons | Spring | Summer | Fall | Winter | Intermediate |
| Organs | Liver, Gall Bladder | Heart, Small Intestine | Lungs, Colon | Kidneys, Bladder | Spleen, Stomach |
| Part Of Body | Tendons, Ligaments | Body Temperature | Bones | Blood | Muscles |
| Fingers | Thumb | Middle Finger | Ring Finger | Little Finger | Index |
| Family | Father's Family | Children | Friends | Relatives | Mother's Family |

The three night divisions and the three humours interact so that:

- 10pm to 1am; phlegm energy increases
- 1am to 4am; bile energy increases
- 4am to 7am; wind energy increases

These energy fluctuations influence our dreams, resulting in people seeing symbols, colours, and experiencing a variety of emotions within dreams. Their meanings also depend on the time that night dreaming takes place. After 7am more unaffected energy circulates, allowing the clarity of prophetic dreams to happen, compared to other times when dreams may appear dull and vague. During the first part of the night, phlegm energy increases our mind, usually reflecting the day's events. So the first part of our sleep is connected with the past.

After midnight the energy of our natural, external environment exerts a stronger influence as nocturnal, non-earthly beings stir, commencing their own cycle. Their energy and powers increase and may influence our mind or even attack our dreams. During this second period strange dreams and nightmares can take place.

During early morning, the third period, our dreams develop clarity as light increases and *rLung* rises within the body. But as the wind energy increases our minds may also destabilise, affecting our dreams accordingly. After seven a.m. the three energies are more balanced and the influence of external energies and disturbances subsides, allowing clearer, prophetic dreams.

Dreams may be classified according to the state of the dreamer - healthy, sick, or the special secret dreams of a skilled practitioner in dream yoga. Generally, dream analysis is based on a person's mental and physical health, useful knowledge to anyone seeking to understand their dreams, not just therapists or doctors.

### Treasure in the Dream
Special or secret dreams belong to the class of uncommon or extraordinary dreams. These dreams are experienced as a result of cultivated practice. The people with these extraordinary dreams are able to manifest the power of their mind. A great master of this is *Dudjom Rinpoche*. In Tibet dream masters called *gTertons* (*Beings who have taken rebirth to uncover the gTerma*) exist with unusual dream abilities, able to realise or access special teachings through their dreams.

However, this power or inherent *siddhi* wisdom lies dormant within each of us, obscured only by our lack of knowledge and negativity. To activate this special ability, mind and energy need to merge. During sleep the possibility of harnessing and tapping into the power of the mind is greater. When asleep our closed eyes shut the sense doors thereby permitting us to concentrate on a large part of our mind. When awake too many thoughts make it difficult to focus the mind. Asleep, we shut down all thinking, making it possible to engage the power of our mind.

If the circulating energy and consciousness are well balanced, the power of mind can be considerably strengthened, no longer distracted by the six sense organs. Closed sense doors provide a greater opportunity for clarity in perception. Even if not embarking on a spiritual practice, clear and prophetic dreams may still be experienced as it is the natural state of our consciousness. If people practise daily to concentrate these parts of their mind they will be able to develop the power of prophetic vision through their dreams. Still, the real power of the mind lies beyond merely the past, present and future.

**Dreaming of the Future**
Prophetic dreams relate to the concept of time. Normally past, present and the future are used as time references, but there are other concepts of time such as summer, winter, watching a flower emerge or saying that this child is growing. Therefore concepts of time are used not just to measure time in a tangible way but in reality these notions of time itself may be questioned. For example, what if time itself does not really exist? When pondered deeply enough, the question may lead to a more profound understanding of what time really means. The easy way out is to say 'I don't understand this.'

We could say that time does not exist. That there is no past, present and future as our consciousness is beyond time and, in saying so, point to the probable nature of prophetic dreams. Based on this rationale, someone should be able to dream exactly what will happen in one year, one month or the next day. Many commonplace examples exist of prophetic dreams. Some prophetic dreams happen exactly as foretold, while others are symbolic in nature. Prophetic dreams coming true will largely depend on the condition of the dreamer's mind, their channels, chakras, breathing and their *rLung*.

The following graph illustrates how prophetic dreams may manifest.

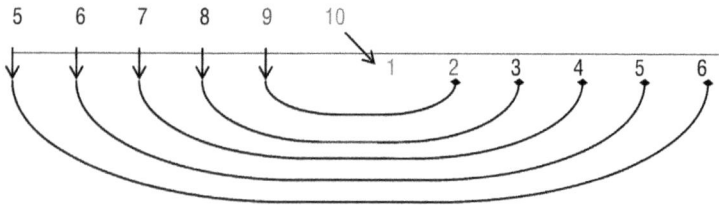

*Illustration of prophetic dreams showing that the earlier the dream occurs, the more likely it will happen further into the future*

Dreams occurring during early morning may reflect the distant future. They may come true perhaps in six days, six months or six years time. On the other hand, late morning dreams (for example 10am) have a better chance of coming true during the day, although logically, 10am could also mean one week, one year, or simply this lifetime. Sequencing dreams reveals the relation between dream and manifestation time.

If consciousness can be considered as the *subject*, time and space would be the *object*. The object can change because of the subject. So mind and consciousness would be the observer, in other words: the mind creates time and space. Depending on the level of consciousness, time and space can therefore manifest in different ways. Logical time and space is connected with our superficial consciousness. The mind experiences realistic space and time through the sense consciousness. But at a deeper or subconscious level, logical time and space can be changed. For instance the speed of dream time is different from that of real time when we are awake. Similarly the notion of space during dream time is different from the waking state. At the level of the base consciousness, which lies beyond the limits of space and time, our mind in that state will be capable of time and space travelling.

## Dreams According to Energy and Typology

The average person's dreams normally relate to their health and according to the typology of the person. In Tibetan medicine the three energies *rLung, mKhris pa, Bad kan* correspond to seven types of people, giving rise to different kinds of dreams. The following table is useful to define each person's energy type (humour).

## Find Your Energy Type – Physical and Personality
Tick those most closely resembling you

| | Physical Test | | |
|---|---|---|---|
| | **Wind** | **Bile** | **Phlegm** |
| **Body Frame** | Small, slender, tall, slender ☐ | Moderate-boned, strong, muscular ☐ | Large, dense-boned, rounded ☐ |
| **Weight** | Thin, tendency to be under-weight ☐ | Moderate ☐ | Overweight or tendency to gain weight easily ☐ |

| | Physical Test | | |
|---|---|---|---|
| | **Wind** | **Bile** | **Phlegm** |
| **Complexion** | Darkish, brownish ☐ | Reddish, yellowish freckles, sensitive to sun ☐ | Fair, pale, white, blemish free ☐ |
| **Skin** | Rough, dry ☐ | Slight oily ☐ | Smooth, thick, oily ☐ |
| **Temperature** | Cold or sensitive to temperature changes ☐ | Warm, hot ☐ | Clammy, cool ☐ |
| **Hair** | Dry, brittle, kinky, normal ☐ | Slightly oily, premature greying or early baldness ☐ | Oily, thick, wavy ☐ |
| **Lips** | Thin ☐ | Moderate ☐ | Thick ☐ |
| **Teeth** | Crooked, oddly shaped ☐ | Moderate size ☐ | Strong, white ☐ |
| **Speech** | Talkative, rapid, ramble ☐ | Precise, sharp, clear ☐ | Slow, monotonous ☐ |
| **Activity** | Very mobile, multi-tasking, likes exercise, dance, moves around ☐ | Moderate, competitive sports ☐ | Little or dislike activity ☐ |
| **Sleep** | Light sleeper, easily wakes ☐ | Moderate ☐ | Deep, sound ☐ |
| **Metabolism** | Changeable digestion ☐ Variable appetite ☐ Feels better after food ☐ | Strong digestion ☐ Big appetite ☐ Easily hungry ☐ Feels better 2-4 hrs after food | Sluggish digestion ☐ Loss of appetite, easily full ☐ Feels better on empty stomach |
| **Total Score** | | | |

| Personality Test | | | | | |
|---|---|---|---|---|---|
| **Intellect** | Fast learner but forgets easily | ☐ | Sharp, intelligent with photographic memory | ☐ | Dull, slow learner but retains information | ☐ |
| **Emotions** | Unstable, changeable | ☐ | Moderate, control | ☐ | Stable, grounded | ☐ |
| | anxious, nervous | ☐ | Anger, aggressive, irritable | ☐ | Depressed, lethargic | ☐ |
| | Insecure, worrying, ambivalent | ☐ | Ambitious | ☐ | Content, satisfied | ☐ |
| **Personality** | Sensitive, creative, fickle, sociable | ☐ | Intense, focus, proud, egotistical, conceited | ☐ | Kind, generous, reliable, sedentary | ☐ |
| Total Score | | | | | |

## The Seven Types of People According to Energy Type

| | |
|---|---|
| *rLung (wind)* | Wind energy is predominant |
| *mKhris pa (bile)* | Bile energy is predominant |
| *Bad kan (phlegm)* | Phlegm energy is predominant |
| *rLung-mKhris pa (wind-bile)* | Wind and bile energy are predominant |
| *mKhris pa-Bad kan (bile-phlegm)* | Bile and phlegm energy are predominant |
| *Bad kan-rLung (phlegm-wind)* | Phlegm and wind energy are predominant |
| *rLung-mKhris pa-Bad kan (wind-bile-phlegm)* | All 3 energies more or less equally dominant |

To analyse dreams in people, the personality type must first be recognised. This is not difficult if we note what colours, symbols and feelings are present in a person's dreams. The dream specific to each type of person as described above can be found in the section 'Meaning of Dreams.'

# Pathological Dreams
# (Warnings in Dreams)

## Health and sleeping position

Generally, dream symbols show good or poor health. People who become ill, such as a person burning with fever, will have very strange colourful dreams; their dreams changing as the fever worsens or abates.

Tibetan medical texts mention dream symbols of sick people usually in terms of energy or circulation blockages in the heart chakra area, which is why we are able to see our problems or illnesses through dreams. The dream symbols belong to the elements, energies and the physical body. The elements are at their most subtle level and so more difficult to understand. For example too much phlegm energy inside in the body will cause a person to dream about rivers, rains or other symbols of water. If someone has heat related problems such as fever (bile problem) their dreams will include hot objects.

Analysing the dreams of sick people must also take into consideration their sleeping position. Not sleeping in the correct position will affect their dreams. When a person has problems with their lungs and heart they might have dreams that someone is pushing down on them, or a heavy object is being pressed on them, or sometimes they might have a sensation of falling.

Dreams like these are associated with sleeping in the wrong position or with hands over the heart. Those who sleep on their stomach or on the left side increase pressure on the heart so that, even when awake, the same pressures can be felt. Whilst sleeping, any pressure around the heart affects the circulation of subtle energies. Therefore, lying on one's back and crossing arms or ankles while trying to sleep creates negative sensations. If a person, especially children, have bad dreams or nightmares, checking their sleeping position would be the first remedy. Sleeping under heavy blankets may also cause troubled sleep.

Pathological dreams usually fall into three categories: (1) physical imbalance, (2) energy imbalance, (3) emotional imbalance.

## Physical Imbalance

### Organs and Their Connections to Dreams
In Tibetan medicine understanding the connection between internal and external organs and their symbolism is crucial in helping to analyse the dream. The **root** (solid) and **flower** (sense) organs, are both linked to special elements.

When an imbalance occurs in the root organs, the dream symbols of the flower organs will produce the symptoms. Therefore, a person with kidney problems can experience hearing changes, or heart issues are shown by a perceptible change in the taste of food and drinks or in the colour of the tongue. Problems with the spleen might show up in different ways such as dry lips or an unhealthy liver through foggy or blurred eyes with a yellow/red tinge and lung problems through the nose, the sense of smell being affected.

If the disorders are strong enough we may become aware that something is wrong. But some people may not display signs of illness and feel merely changes in their energy levels and their sense bases. Having body odours may also mean a lung or nose disorder. As our nervous system and heart is tied to our breathing, problems here are seen as breathing difficulties and heart palpitations.

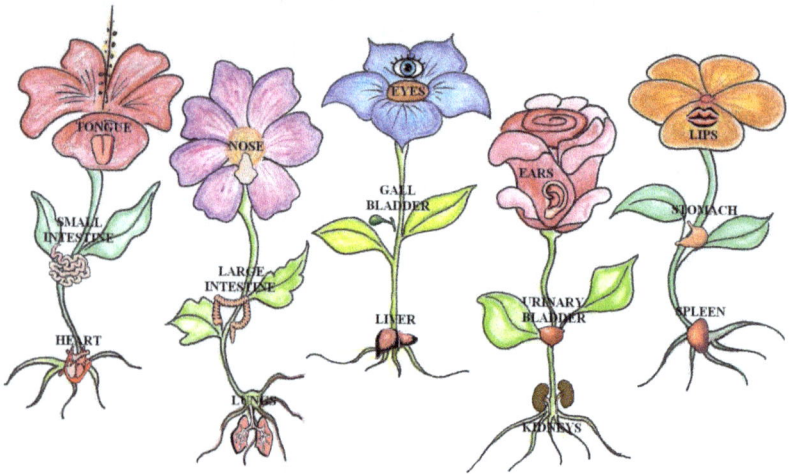

### Relationship between Seasons and Organs

| Seasons | Spring | Summer | Autumn | Winter | Transition |
|---------|--------|--------|--------|--------|------------|
| Organs | Liver | Heart | Lungs | Kidneys | Spleen |
| | Gall bladder | Small intestines | Colon | Urinary bladder | Stomach |
| | Eyes | Tongue | Nose | Genital organs | Lips |
| | | | | Ears | Skin |
| Elements | Wood | Fire | Metal | Water | Earth |

## Element Table

| Dimension | | | | | | |
|---|---|---|---|---|---|---|
| **Subtle** | **Origin of elements** | sound → | | light → | rays → | |
| | Subtle anatomy | Vajra mind | | Vajra voice | Vajra body | |
| | Emotions | unaware | desire | anger, pride, jealousy | ignorance | delusion |
| **Gross** | **Internal elements** | space → | wind → | fire → | water → | earth |
| | Creation of body | emptiness | movement | speed | liquid | solidity |
| | Senses | hearing | touch | seeing | tasting | smelling |
| | Solid organs (From pure part) | heart | lungs | liver | kidneys | spleen |
| | Hollow organs (From impure part) | small bowel | large bowel | gall bladder | urinary bladder, genital organs | stomach |
| | Body function | body cavities | breathing | complexion | blood, lymph | bones, tendons |
| | Body parts | head | right leg | right arm | left leg | left arm |
| | **External elements** | fire | metal | wood | water | earth |
| | Sense organs | tongue | nose | eyes | ears | lips |
| | Seasons | summer | autumn | spring | winter | intersection |

These simple examples illustrate how Tibetan medicine analyses the different physical problems or energy imbalances, at variance from western medical science. To understand the meaning of dreams in Tibetan medicine we must comprehend the relationship between the senses (colours, smells, sounds, touch and taste) and the functions of the internal organs (heart, lungs, liver, kidneys, spleen); the elements (earth, water, fire, wind, and space); the four seasons and the humours (*rLung, mKhris pa, Bad kan*). This knowledge is fundamental in successfully diagnosing a disease.

Any worries about health or perceived danger or threats to one's life is revealed through dream symbols as worries are just suppressed fears working at a subconscious level and emerging symbolically in dreams.

## ENERGY IMBALANCE

### *bLa* Energy

A special energy called *bLa* (ཨ), circulates within the body at a gross level, and at a subtler level moves with the mind or consciousness. If a dying person has a very strong attachment for another, an animal, or even an object, this emotion or energy can remain in that place or with the object after death. Just like a bowl of garlic taken out of a room leaves a residual smell after it is gone.

When consciousness leaves the body at the moment of death, it is possible for the energy to remain and, if very negative, to attack another person. This sort of attack may be difficult to sense while we are awake. It can however be experienced quite clearly in our dreams where the subtle energies move easily from one person to another. A person's mind may also affect another's dreams through the subtle energies of thoughts, able to influence your dreams just as you can affect theirs. If a person is performing black magic and their actions are aimed at being deliberately injurious to others, or their thoughts detrimental, special dream symbols may appear. The *bLa* energy's monthly cycle is strongly connected to lunar energy moving throughout the body including the toes.

| Cycle of solar energy | Cycle of lunar energy |
|---|---|
| *7-10 am* | *Sunset* |
| base chakra active, rising red energy gives happiness | head chakra active, feeling fearful, lunar energy like melting ice |
| *10 am-12 pm* | *Stars shining* |
| navel chakra active, warming up creates desire | 16 drops fall from 1st to 2nd chakra (1 for each petal of 2nd chakra) |
| *12-2 pm* | *Midnight* |
| heart chakra active, mind becomes heavier | 8 drops fall into 3rd chakra, 8 drops dissolve in body |
| *2-5 pm* | *After midnight* |
| throat chakra active, mind is more emotional - sadness, arguments, quarrels | 4 drops fall into 4th chakra, 4 drops dissolve in body |
| *5 pm* | *Early morning* |
| head chakra active, sunset | 2 drops fall into 5th chakra, 2 drops dissolve in body, last 2 drops dissolve into red energy |

Up to the age of 25 solar, but predominantly lunar energy, increase within each person. Both energies, particularly solar, then stabilise between 25 and 45, after which they decrease, with solar weakening.

## Path of *bLa*

*bLa* energy takes a different path in men and women: the male cycle starting at the left leg, ascending to the top and then down the right leg. In the female, *bLa* starts at the right leg, travelling up before descending the left leg. Lunar energy starts from the big toe on the first day of the waxing moon, every day moving up a little until it reaches the crown at full moon. During full moon people generally are more sensitive as the entire body fills with lunar energy like a bottle filled with light. From the new moon onwards, the peaceful lunar energy of *Yar Ngo* (upper facing moon) grows, accumulating each day with its corresponding peace aspects. However as the full moon wanes, *Mar Ngo* energy (down facing moon) takes over, the peaceful aspect of Mar Mo energy decreasing with the rise of the former.

With weakening moon energy, the wrathful aspect of solar energy grows so that on the 30th day, with the lunar energy having completed a full cycle ending at the soles of the feet, solar power is now located at the crown. On the first day of the new moon, lunar energy is once again absorbed into the toe. Therefore when lunar energy ascends on one side, solar energy descends on the other, the direction being opposite for male and female. When the body is full of lunar energy, solar energy located at our soles is weak. But when solar energy rises to the top and the lunar energy is at the bottom, everything becomes more chaotic. So, during *yar ngo*, first half of the month, people generally feel greater peace and happiness, their cycle occupied by lunar energy. But during mar ngo when solar energy is more active, people are easily emotional and depressed.

According to Tibetan astrology, based on the lunar calendar, the 1ˢᵗ – 15ᵗʰ of each month is the peaceful period, and the rest of the month from the 16ᵗʰ – 30ᵗʰ marks the wrathful time. Hence, peaceful deity practices are done in the first half of the month and wrathful deity practices in the second. For this reason some Tibetan masters prefer going into a cave retreat during the wrathful period and are only active during half the month. The wrathful period is also the time of obstacles. In *Yuthok Nyingthig* it is mentioned that *Yuthok* practice should be started in the first half of the month, if peaceful results are desired. Therefore soft therapies are preferred during the first 15 days, while rough therapies like bloodletting and moxa are encouraged in the second half. During the full and new moon it's best to avoid rough, invasive therapies such as operations or teeth extraction, *bLa* energy being also easily lost through acupuncture needles. The easiest entry points for bLa energy come from the ring fingers and toes. Blocking these points traps the *bLa* energy within, preventing its loss.

When solar and lunar energy are well balanced, the body is healthy. Imbalance of these internal energies leads to obstacles in life. *Vajrayana* practitioners do exercises to balance solar and lunar energies for health reasons and to avoid spiritual obstacles. Natural protectors called དག་ར་ལྷ་ *dgra lha* reside within the body.

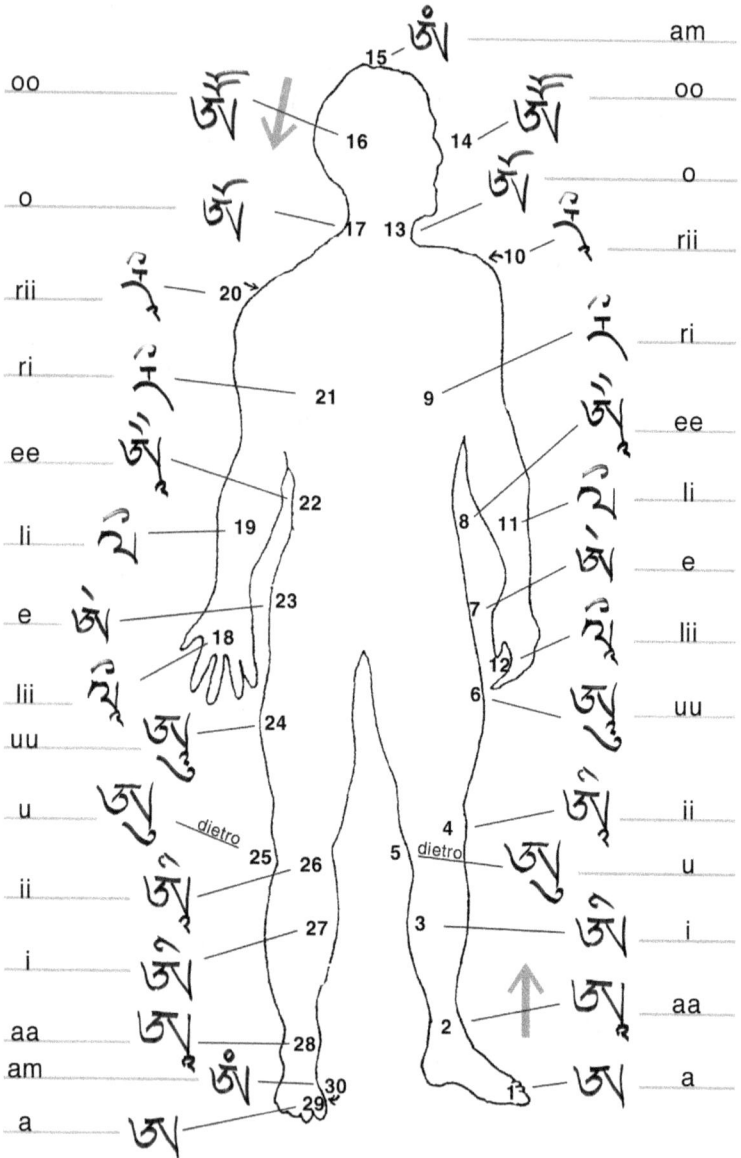

*Path of bLa in The Body*

## *rLung* and Dreams

Subtle *rLung* is always connected to mind or consciousness and when this energy is seriously weakened, it is unable to function at a physical level. Despite this, even a person with weak *rLung*, thinking about someone either positively or negatively, will be able to exert an influence on others through a subtle projection of their thoughts.

Imbalances from the three humours affect the digestion system:

| Part of digestion system | Humours |
| --- | --- |
| Stomach | Phlegm |
| Duodenum, small intestine | Bile |
| Colon | Wind |

Improper food can cause unbalanced dreams.

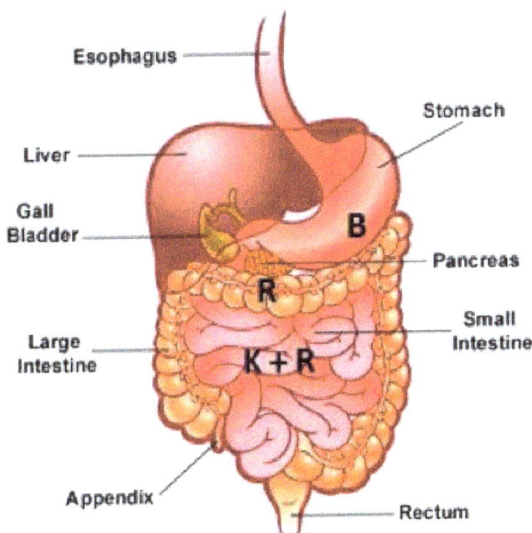

79

# EMOTIONAL IMBALANCES

## Knots

Emotional pathological dreams generally refer to all negative feelings troubling people. According to Tibetan dream teachers, the mind is like a rope with many knots, each, expressing a disturbed feeling or emotion.

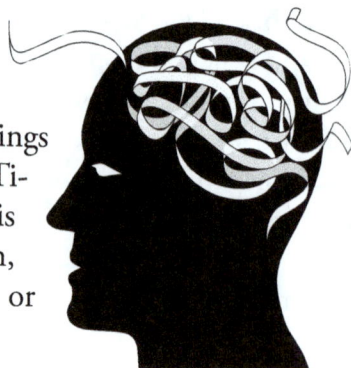

©JP Chiaverio 2013

## Knots of Disturbed Feelings

1. Fear
2. Panic
3. Anger
4. Hatred
5. Sadness
6. Grief
7. Frustration
8. Anxiety
9. Worry
10. Confusion
11. Helplessness
12. Desperation
13. Feeling incapable
14. Disability
15. Insensitivity
16. Jealousy
17. Embarrassment
18. Conflict
19. Regret
20. Homesick
21. Separation
22. Manipulation
23. Shock
24. Depression
25. Abandonment
26. Lost
27. Trapped
28. Pain
29. Stress
30. Out of control
31. Phobia
32. Loneliness
33. Humiliation
34. Rejection
35. Dissatisfaction
36. Unhappiness
37. Lethargy
38. Rage
39. Impotence
40. Intolerance
41. Devalued
42. Disappointment
43. Disorientation
44. Numbness
45. Madness
46. Manic
47. Guilt
48. Craving
49. Upset
50. Annoyance

## Warnings

Dreams can provide warnings of life threatening disorders. According to the *Four Medical Tantras* a dream can clearly show when there is the threat of imminent danger to a person's life. Therefore dreams may be important predictions of an onset of illness before it actually happens.

| Warning Dreams | | Meaning |
|---|---|---|
| Riding a cat, monkey, tiger, fox, or a corpse | → | ensnared by *Yama* |
| Riding a buffalo, horse, pig, donkey or camel while naked and heading south | → | indicates death |
| Willow tree with bird's nest growing from one's head | → | under control of *Yama* |
| Palmyra or other thorny trees growing from one's heart | → | under control of *Yama* |
| Removing a lotus from one's heart | → | *Yama* |
| Falling down a precipice | → | *Yama* |
| Sleeping in a cemetery | → | *Yama* |
| Injury to one's head | → | *Yama* |
| Encircled by crows, hungry ghosts | → | *Yama* |
| Person of low birth | → | *Yama* |
| Skin falling off own limbs | → | *Yama* |
| Entering back into mother's womb | → | *Yama* |
| Drowning, falling into quicksand | → | *Yama* |
| Swallowed by a fish | → | *Yama* |
| Finding abundant iron/gold/money | → | *Yama* |
| Loss in business transactions or arguments | → | *Yama* |
| Pursued for payment of food / entertainment | → | *Yama* |
| Fetching a bride | → | *Yama* |
| Naked | → | *Yama* |
| Cutting hair or shaving one's beard | → | *Yama* |
| Drinking a toast with deceased relatives | → | *Yama* |
| Dragged by deceased relatives | → | *Yama* |

| Warning Dreams | Meaning |
|---|---|
| Wearing a dress or ornament with red colour → | *Yama* |
| Dancing with deceased relatives → | *Yama* |
| Dreaming of Gods, leaders of herds, holy people, famous people → | longevity, health, prosperity |
| Blazing fire, sea → | longevity, health, prosperity |
| One's body smeared with blood and filth → | longevity, health prosperity |
| Wearing white clothes → | longevity, health prosperity |
| Hoisting *Phen* or *Dug* and obtaining fruits → | longevity, health prosperity |
| Climbing a high mountain or roof top of a beautiful building → | positive result |
| A fruit laden tree → | positive result |
| Riding lion, elephant, horse, cow or ox → | positive result |
| Crossing a wide river or sea, heading north or east → | positive result |
| Escaping from miserable conditions → | positive result |
| Defeating one's enemies → | positive result |
| Receiving praise and veneration from parents or deities → | positive result |

# Classification of Dreams

## Healthy and Unhealthy Dreams

Dreams can be classified according to different systems. The Four Tantra Classifications of Dreams include Healthy and Unhealthy Dreams:

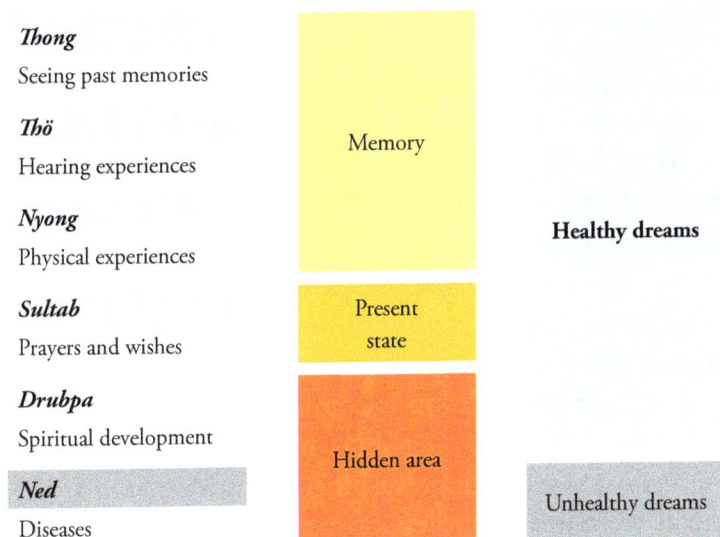

**Thong**
Seeing past memories

**Thö**
Hearing experiences

**Nyong**
Physical experiences

**Sultab**
Prayers and wishes

**Drubpa**
Spiritual development

**Ned**
Diseases

Memory

Present state

Hidden area

**Healthy dreams**

Unhealthy dreams

Dream phenomena can be further classified according to past, present and future.

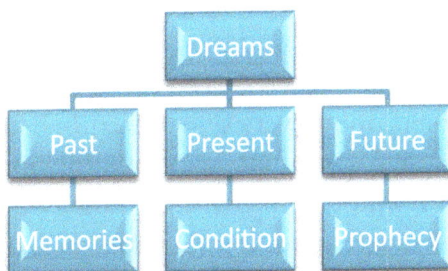

Dreams
- Past — Memories
- Present — Condition
- Future — Prophecy

# Symbols – Language of Dreams

In dream analysis dream symbols are considered carefully. Dreams contain a wide variety of symbols that show our current state of health. In Buddhist culture and philosophy, symbolism plays a constant role in daily life, as well as in dreams as everything is perceived to be interdependent.

Dream symbols take on significant meanings when their importance is studied and understood. All the ancient religions whether Buddhist, Christian, Judaic or Bön, attach various symbols to different objects. So based on nationality, culture, subculture or even the difference between one person and the next, symbols always existed bearing their own special meanings.

From a greater perspective, there is no difference between nations, cultures, or people with their individual biases, as the basic human condition is commonly shared. Thus underlying symbolic meanings may be similar. For example, water is used for drinking, washing, swimming or sports by virtually everyone regardless of national or cultural differences. In this respect, we all share a common understanding or attitude towards water. Even if many objects and rituals exist within their own cultural context, the common understanding is there (yaks are found only in Tibet and a Tibetan may dream of yak dung, while a Westerner dreams of cow dung. The point is, dung is dung!).

In Tibetan philosophy, every object used in daily life and its attributes takes on a symbolic meaning, including its name, form, function and colour, which means symbolic dreams can be readily understood. It might appear that dream symbols have a personal or cultural significance, but their true meaning go far beyond the constraints of personal and cultural interpretations.

Dream symbols we refer to are therefore universal symbols with meanings similar to all cultures. Usually they appear as:
- Positive dream symbols with positive meanings
- Positive dream symbols with negative meanings
- Negative dream symbols with positive meanings
- Negative dream symbols with negative meanings

*A list of symbols and their meanings can be found in the section 'Meaning of Dreams.'*

Until now we have only looked at dream symbols as a reflection of daily life experiences. However it is equally important to note that planetary influences affect our dreams just as much as the immediate environment, whether through ethereal beings or other external causes.

Not all dream symbols are portents of meaning. Many merely reflect mundane details of daily life and past experiences. To know if a dream is prophetic in nature, only study, practice and experience will allow one to discern the difference between reflective, symbolic and prophetic dreams. When interpreting dreams, the season must be considered, followed by a person's sleeping position, and what he or she has been doing. The dream interpreter has to listen carefully to the dream being told and try to understand the dreamer's relationships with other people before starting to analyse the dream.

In reflective dreams, symbols only occupy a small part of the dream. For example, if I dream I am talking to you within a group, and I suddenly see a hat, my attention immediately switching back to the group, my dream is a reflection of my experiences with the hat symbol being one small part of the dream. Not all dreams are symbolic and it is difficult to figure if a particular object is indeed of symbolic significance. However, if an element or something in a dream stands out clearly, and is remembered with strong clarity during waking time, then that part of the dream would most likely be symbolic.

In Tibetan culture bad dreams are talked about to diminish their power and good dreams are kept secret to empower their potential. Talking about dream symbols inhibits their power. To cleanse and disempower a negative dream, recite a purification mantra like *Vajrasattva*, a Buddha or deity mantra such as *Simhamukha*, Green Tara or *Padmasambhava*.

## How to Analyse a Dream

Start by seeing a dream as a movie. Then proceed to cut and edit the film according to the different dream classifications. This method is similar to anatomical study, whereby we completely cut open the dream to analyse it bit by bit. This technique helps understand dreams. The following table shows how this is done:

| Dream parts | Location | Figure 1 | Figure 2 | Figure 3 | Situation | Emotion | Object | Time |
|---|---|---|---|---|---|---|---|---|
| Analysis | Memory | Present condition | Unknown | Memory | Desire | Desire | Unknown | Morning |

According to this table we need to analyse the unknown parts so we can understand the full meaning of a dream. For psychological issues the memories are important too. Some dreams are simple dreams - just a memory or a present desire which is easy to analyse or understand. Some dreams are very mixed - a combination of memory, present condition and prophetic dream parts. These dreams, referred to as 'cocktail dreams', may take longer and require more effort to interpret.

## Example: A symbolic dream?

A Tibetan girl living in Rome had a dream very early one morning around 4 or 5am. In her dream, she was in Tibet and it was snowing heavily, and everything was covered by it. She saw her grandfather, a very old man, climbing up the stairs leading to the roof of a Tibetan style of house. She saw her grandfather fall and cried out. Upon waking she had real tears and felt really sad.

This kind of dream might appear symbolic. but in reality it isn't. The images of snow, the grandfather, stairs, and the Tibetan house may seem like symbols but they are the result of the girl's past experiences. In Tibet she had lived in a similar type of house, and when each winter it started her grandfather climbed the stairs to clean the snow from the roof. And each time she worried about her grandfather doing this. The dream here is clearly reflective - the house, the grandfather, the stairs and the snow (even if her grandfather still continues to climb the stairs and will most likely do so in the future) indicate a possibility that this may also be a prophetic dream.

When she related this dream during a workshop I conducted in Italy, I thought the dream was highly unlikely to be symbolic, especially after probing for details of her life in Tibet. Listening to her story I could see that her dream images were commonplace occurrences linked with her daily life in Tibet. Since I was concerned that she might infer this to be a prophetic dream, I told her in all likelihood that it was merely a reflective type of dream.

## Checklist for Dream Analysis

Carefully following this checklist will help analyse dreams.

1. Note the season and the stage of that season in the dream, for example, is it early winter or late autumn?
2. Link this to the five external elements.
3. Check the sleeping position and whether heavy blankets are used which can affect sleep and dream quality.
4. Ask questions about work, family, work or social relationships, including everyday experiences to know more about a person's daily routine.
5. Listen carefully to what they feel is important to them.
6. Listen to their dream keeping in mind what they have already told you. If there is something that stands out or seems an odd part of the dream, yet stays very clear in a person's memory then that part of the dream would most likely be symbolic in nature.
7. Check the time of the person's dream and relate this to a dream's timelines and the corresponding humour.
8. Ask about the colours in the dream.
9. Find out how the person felt when he/she first woke up; were the residual feelings pleasant, unpleasant or neutral?
10. Identify the person's energy typology.
11. Explain why you think the dream was either reflective, symbolic or prophetic.
12. If possible, keep in touch with the person to hear about further dreams or if consequences developed from the dream.

The more we work with dreams, the more everything appears symbolic! It is therefore crucial to check day time experiences and carefully connect those experiences with what is happening in the dreams.

Being committed to dream practice, and regularly analysing dreams is important for anyone seeking to become an adept in the Tibetan art of dream analysis. A beginner wanting to study Tibetan dream analysis would be expected to commence basic homework by starting with the interpretation of ten dreams, just to become familiar with the concepts of Tibetan dream cosmology. Proficiency in understanding and interpreting Tibetan dream analysis only develops when all the dream symbols are fully understood and the interpreter is able to discern accurately between reflective or prophetic dreams.

# Part Two

# Dream Analysis Techniques

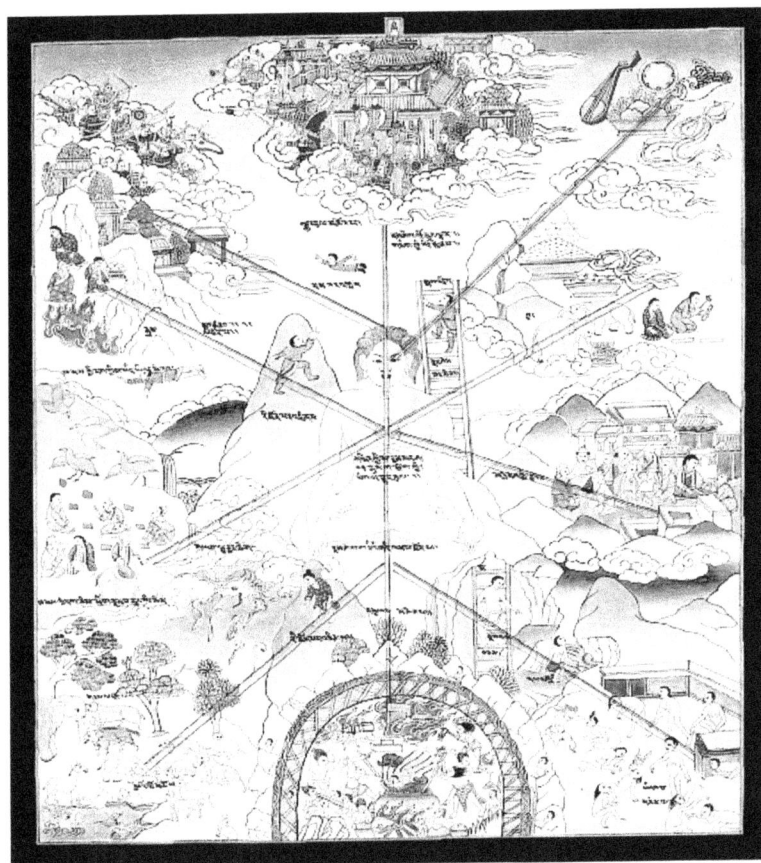

# Overview

According to Tibetan tradition there are three methods of dream analysis or dream studies:
- Dream Work
- Dream Practice
- Dream Yoga

**Dream work** is a medical approach emphasizing the release of blocked emotions which can cause diseases.

**Dream practice** comes from the Shamanic tradition. The aims are to enhance lucid dreaming, prophetic dreaming, clairvoyance and divination.

**Dream yoga** arises from the *Vajrayana* approach, where the ultimate objective of the practice is Self-Realisation (Total Awareness).

## Dream Work

### Unblocking Disturbed Emotions
Dream work consists of a series of mental exercises to reach the dream state in order to create a change, and heal an existing imbalance. Our mind, emotions and subtle channels appear like a rope which can become entangled into multiple knots. Dream work seeks to untie these knots.

Therefore dream work helps to:
- Unblock energetic channels
- Release blocked emotions

- Prevent and remove stress and tension
- Tone organs

The mental techniques shown involve acting out dreams while staying in the two states of Perfect (total) Self-Acceptance and Self-Confidence. These exercises can be developed either through group training or working alone.

**The Two Mental Exercises of Dream Work**

| (Perfect) Self-Acceptance | (Perfect) Self-Confidence |
|---|---|
| Accept that emotions are natural, not allowing the mind's logic to reject what you may feel. | Knowing that Self is the creator of the dream dimension, provides the capacity to create or change dreams and circumstances. |

## Acting Out in Group Work

Dream practice can take place either among a group of participants, or a session conducted between the dream healer and the dreamer. There are five main steps to observe:

## Step 1
The dreamer is in a comfortable, relaxed position, either sitting or lying down. The dreamer takes a deep breath, visualising the body as totally empty with only the three channels present.

## Step 2
Before beginning the dream, the dreamer has to choose either a disturbing or habitually unpleasant dream, before dropping into a state of deep relaxation, or falling asleep. If there is a difficulty in choosing a dream, focus instead on an annoying incident or an emotional upheaval encountered recently or present in everyday life.

### Step 3
The dream healer, working with the dream story, encourages the dreamer to intensify the dream experience through vivid, guided visualisation techniques intensifying the emotions felt without undue exaggeration.

### Step 4
As the dream grows in intensity through the senses being tuned up (sight, hearing, smell, touch or taste) the dreamer is helped by unblocking the emotional content and releasing it.

### Step 5
The dream session ends with the dreamer relaxing, breathing deeply and being fully aware that everything that took place happened only in the dream world, and was merely an illusion. A realisation that even in highly disturbing dreams, nothing harmful took place.

> **Caution:** This dream visualisation technique should not be practised with people who suffer from **heart disease**, **high blood pressure**, or are **overly emotional** or **hypersensitive**.

It is important to periodically check a dreamer's heartbeat, and if at any time someone becomes too emotionally wrought, the practice should end immediately.

### Acting Out with Self-Training
Self-training or working alone in dream practice can be considered as a meditative practice.

**Step 1**

Sit or lie down in a very relaxed position, breathing deeply either through the nose or mouth.

**Step 2**

As with group practice, visualise the body as empty, containing only the three channels, with the *rLung* energy moving from the navel chakra to the heart chakra. When it reaches this point, drop deeply into sleep, starting from the throat chakra, to begin the dream.

**Step 3**

Strongly visualising the dream, try to create the disturbing emotion or emotions felt during the dream.

**Step 4**

Unblock the disturbing emotion by choosing either the empowerment of perfect self-confidence or self-acceptance, whichever choice works better.

**Step 5**

Release or end the dream experience, allowing everything that has been experienced during the process to go to a place of deep peace. Relax, and finish off with a deep breath.

If a feeling threatens to overwhelm you during the process, opening the eyes is a reassuring measure to remind you that you are safe, and what is being experienced is only a mental exercise.

## Chart showing emotions, their respective energy and channel blockages, and choice of dream work technique

| Emotion | Blockage | Solution |
|---|---|---|
| Anxiety<br>Confusion<br>Fear<br>Panic<br>Phobia<br>Stress<br>Worry | Energy and channels | Perfect Self-Confidence |
| Feeling Abandoned<br>Frustration<br>Grief<br>Homesickness<br>Sadness<br>Separation/Loneliness<br>Unhappiness | Energy | Perfect Self-Acceptance |
| Depression<br>Disability<br>Helplessness Hopelessness<br>Impotence<br>Powerlessness<br>Senselessness | Energy and channels | Perfect Self-Confidence |
| Conflict/ Manipulation<br>Embarrassment | Energy and channels | Perfect Self-Confidence |
| Lost<br>Pain<br>Regret<br>Shock<br>Trapped Humiliation | Energy | Perfect Self-Acceptance |
| Anger<br>Craving<br>Hatred<br>Jealousy<br>Out of control | Energy | Perfect Self-Acceptance |

| Emotion | Blockage | Solution |
|---------|----------|----------|
| Annoyance Guilt Madness Manic Numbness Upset | Energy and channels | Perfect Self-Confidence |
| Intolerance Lethargy Rage Rejection Devalued | Energy and channels | Perfect Self-Confidence |
| Disappointment Dissatisfaction Disoriented | Energy and channels | Perfect Self-Acceptance |

# Dream Practice

## Methods of Dream Practice

Dream Practice is an ancient method of manipulating dreams which originates from the shamanic tradition. Abilities such as lucid dreaming, prophetic dreaming, clairvoyance, and divination can be developed and improved through practice. By using visualisation techniques the mind is also trained in meditation and prepared for the practice of Dream Yoga.

The Dream Practice consists of a combined knowledge of astrology, the recitation of mantras and the art of visualisation.

**Dream Practice**

| Astrology | Mantra Recitations | Visualisation |
|-----------|--------------------|--------------| 
| Considers dates that are most appropriate for specific practices, together with the most propitious planetary influences | Working with sound. The vibrations create the setting to realise the mind's true potential | Crystal practice. Can be done as sleep practice before reciting mantras |

### Crystal Practice (lucid dreaming)

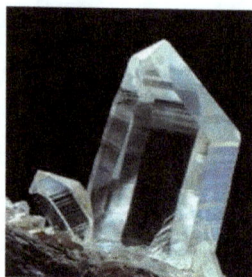

#### *Step 1 Memorise a crystal*
Start by looking at a crystal and memorising it. The image you see should be as clear as possible. In the beginning your images may be hazy, or unstable. However, looking at a crystal or a clear glass of water for 15 minutes before sleeping can help to create a clear picture in your memory. Keep in your mind's eye the three qualities of a crystal: pure, clear and limpid.

#### *Step 2 Visualise your brain or head as a crystal*
Try to imagine your entire brain as made of crystal and, contained within a crystal head, your eyes, ears, nose, mouth, skin and hair are equally clear and transparent.

#### *Step 3 Visualise your entire body as a single crystal*
Imagine your body as a single piece of clear crystal. Leave out of your visualisation details of the limbs or torso of the body.

#### *Step 4 Visualise a single eye on your crystal body*

#### *Step 5 Visualise the entire crystal of your body covered by countless eyes*
During this five-step visualisation process, proceed only to the next step if a visualisation image is stable. For any difficulty in visualisation encountered at any specific step, this should be practised until a clear picture emerges in the mind before moving on. After five weeks of daily crystal practice for 15 minutes, you should be able to notice the first changes resulting from your practice in lucid dreaming.

## Dream Yoga

The first medical book that mentions dream yoga in the Tibetan medical tradition, *Yuthok Nyingthig*, refers to it as one of the Six Types of Yoga, namely Divine Fire, Clear Light, Transferring Consciousness, Illusory Body, Dream and Bardo Yoga.

Dream Yoga, also called sleeping meditation, is one of the most important schools of mind study in the Tibetan *Vajrayana* tradition. In dream yoga, mental exercises are used to develop the capacity of the mind by way of the subtle *rLung* energy. Through the practice of dream yoga, one reaches a real understanding of self and becomes aware of the true nature of the mind. Thus lucid dreaming and meditation exercises lead to self knowledge.

Once we are able to understand and develop our ability in dream yoga, our view on life and death changes, as expressed in the diagram here showing the Dream Yoga Division.

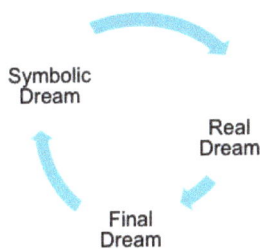

Symbolic
Dream

Real
Dream

Final
Dream

Symbolic dream carries its own logic, which is as equally important as the logic used in daily life. In fact, Tibetan dream doctors consider life to be an illusory dream – the actual, 'real dream' more illusionary than even dreaming, as the illusion is harder to perceive. And the final dream is referred to as **illusionary death**.

Visualisation of the centre of throat chakra - *Amitabha* with consort on the lotus

[part 2 of the Dream Yoga text next page]

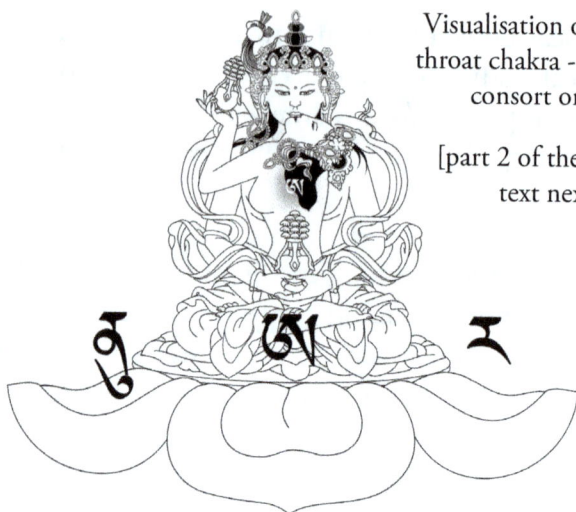

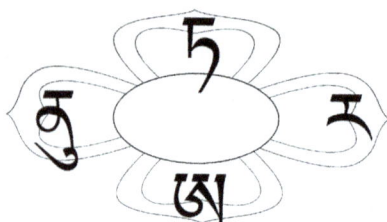

Lotus upon which one visualises the centre of the throat chakra - *Amitabha* with consort

| | |
|---|---|
| | A |
| | NU |
| | TA |
| | RA |

The letters can be of any preferred colour, with the exception of A, located in the heart of *Amitabha*, which is coral red

*The following text can only be truly followed*
*if a person has received transmission*

## From the Original Dream Yoga Text
## in the Yuthok Nyingthig (གཡུ་ཐོག་སྙིང་ཐིག་གི་རྨི་ལམ་རྣལ་འབྱོར)

Dream Yoga, the Self-Purifying Illusion (*rmi lam nying krul rang dag* (རྨི་ལམ་ཉིང་འཁྲུལ་རང་དག))

## Part 1 Day Practice
During the day, while eating, dressing, walking, sitting, sleeping, or at any moment in your life, imagine the following: "I'm sleeping" and "I'm dreaming". Think of all that is happening as a dream and an illusion. *And say this aloud.*

## Part 2 Practice Before Falling Asleep
Before sleeping, visualise at the centre of the throat chakra a white lotus flower with four petals. Your primordial awareness arises as *Guru Amitabha* in union[1], one *tson*[2] in size. In his heart there is a coral-coloured A ཨ. On the four petals stand the four syllables - *A Nu Ta Ra* ཨ་ནུ་ཏ་ར་ – (visualise this in a colour of your choice). *Amitabha's* consort is offering him great bliss (*see image on page 100*).

*May I be able to catch the dream,*
*To realize my own awareness within the dream,*
*To transform the dream,*
*To avoid fear in the dream,*
*And to understand the truth of the dream.*

After you recite the prayer, [and while chanting the mantra *OM A NU TA RA]*, visualise that red light to be like the

---

1 The primordial awareness is represented by *Guru Amitabha,* united with his consort
2 A tson = two fingers. The union of the Guru and his consort being this size

rising sun radiating from the body of the guru, eliminating from your body all bad karma and provocations. Your body fills with red light which then expands beyond your body. All of space becomes *pure land* and all sentient beings become dakas and dakinis. The light is offered to all buddhas and bodhisattvas. The light comes back to the guru's heart and the *A* becomes very radiant and colourful. Focus your mind on it, [with as much concentration] as if you were threading a needle.

Just before falling asleep remind yourself [verbally or mentally] 21 times to catch your dream.

## Part 3  Catching the dream

If you fall asleep mindfully, you can catch the dream[3]. If you cannot catch it, it is because of your weak devotion and thick bad karma, and your lack of desire, courage and effort. Be more mindful and pray more from your inner heart. If you still cannot catch the dream after repeating this[4] a few times, visualise your guru in your head, heart, navel or base chakra[5].

Upon waking, if you succeeded in catching your dream, do not open your eyes; keep them closed, while being mindful and relaxed. This will help you further in overcoming the difficulty of catching your dream.[6]

## Part 4  Transforming the Dream

Once you have a stable base from which to catch your dreams regularly, you should do purification, multiplication and transformation. You will then be able to catch

---

3 Meaning you will dream lucidly
4 Visualisation of the guru at your throat
5 Meaning try visualisation at other chakras one at a time to see which brings a result
6 Opening your eyes will distract you

your dream at any time you wish, and your dream practice becomes stable.

During the day[7], imagine yourself in a dream and that you need to transform all experiences[8]. That within the dream the dream fire does not burn you, nor dream water floods you, neither can you fall off a dream cliff. Imagine yourself to be totally free of all restrictions in whatever you choose to do. Do the same meditation with wild animals and evil spirits (dream animals cannot attack, nor dream spirits harm). Practise this constantly.

Invoke these meditative thoughts constantly before falling asleep. When you succeed in catching your dream, repeat the same actions during the day. For example, if you imagine an animal attacking you during the day, strongly accompany the image with, "this is a dream animal and therefore cannot attack or harm me". Then when you see an animal while dreaming, the result will be exactly the same.

During the day, in whatever you see or experience, think of it as a dream. And in that dream you can do anything. Like transforming water into fire, and fire into water. Or able to change and multiply objects at will, whether a hundred or a thousand times. If you see sentient beings, imagine they are your deity, again multiplying their numbers from one to infinity.

## Antidotes

If you encounter demons in your dream[9], you can subdue them by invoking various, stronger, more powerful anti-

---

7 As part of meditation
8 Experiences you desire to transform
9 For example as a negative feeling, presence, or odour

dotes (opponents). For *Gyelpo* spirits visualise yourself as *Hayagriva*. for *Za, Vajrapani*, and for *Nagas, Nagaraksha*.

In the same way if you encounter a dog, see a wolf. For a wolf see a tiger, and for the tiger, a lion. You can therefore visualise a stronger animal to conquer the previous one.

## Pure Land

You can also visit any pure land you wish, to listen to any Buddha's teachings, ride the sun and moon to visit the four continents, or if you desire to visit someone, or transform into a bird. If your dream is still unclear, you must be more mindful before sleeping. Focus the mind strongly.[10] Repeating the pure land visualisation many times will slowly make the mind clearer. Eventually you will succeed.

*The following text can only be truly followed*
*if a person has received transmission*

## Yoga Practice

If you catch the dream but the ability to transform it remains weak, your *rLung* energy is weak. This can be offset by practicing *bum ba chen*. When you visualise the navel chakra, *rLung* and consciousness must be strongly held there [mentally]. If you cannot enter into earth within the dream, then during dream yoga practice you must lower your energy [from the navel]. If you can't fly within your dream it means your *rLung* and consciousness have to be raised [from the navel]. If you are unable to fly horizontally, direct your energy and consciousness in that specific direction.

---

10 Visualising the throat chakra guru

# Preparation for Dream Practice

## 1 Location
- Quiet, such as countryside, preferably without a pet
- Normal temperature, neither too hot or cold
- Dark place; not too much light
- No obstacles or activities during the retreat

## 2 Mind and body
- Relaxation and rest for both body and mind. No work or worry.
- Yoga and movement allowed
- No newspapers, novels, etc.
- No TV, and as little radio as possible
- No mobile phones or internet

## 3 Food
- Light food, such as soup, cooked vegetables. Heavy food affects digestion and dreaming
- Reduce fluid intake, as too much can affect dreams
- No alcohol, drugs, vitamins or soft drinks
- No coffee or tea, as these can cause insomnia and affect dream work

## 4 Timing
- Any time during the day
- Before sleep
- During sleep

## Starting The Actual Practice of Dream Yoga

Before sleep, purify your breathing with the following breathing exercises while adopting the seven pointed postures of *Vairocana* as shown below.

### The Seven Meditation Postures of *Vairocana*

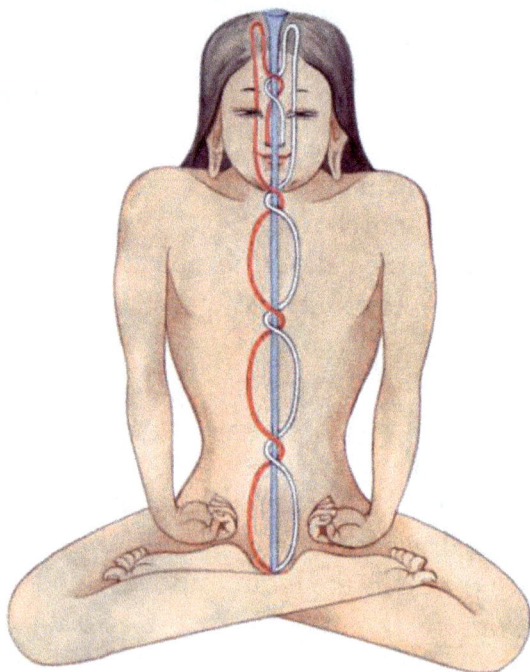

1. Sit cross-legged. Ideally in full lotus position.
   Balances descending wind
2. Keep the spine straight.
   Balances fire-accompanying wind
3. Clasp the hands in *vajra* fists pressing on the groin.
   Balances descending wind
4. Press the tongue to the palate, just behind the teeth.
   Balances life-sustaining wind

5. Lift the shoulders with straightened arms, like a folded eagle's wings.
   Balances all-pervading wind
6. The chin should be slightly tucked in, like a swan.
   Balances ascending wind
7. Gaze at the tip of the nose, or just beyond.
   Balances life-sustaining wind

## The Three Channels in Purification Breathing
The three channels, their colours and their characteristics

| Right Channel<br>རོ་མ roma | Central Channel<br>དབུ་མ uma | Left Channel<br>རྐྱང་མ kyangma |
|---|---|---|
| Anger/Hatred | Attachment/Desire | Ignorance/Delusion |
| Fire | Wind | Water and Earth |
| Red | Blue | White |
| Solar | Neutral | Lunar |
| Bile | Wind | Phlegm |
| Snake | Rooster | Pig |

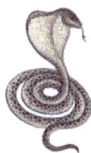

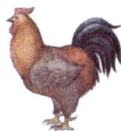

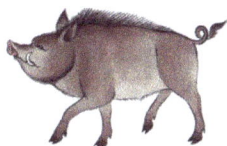

## The Nine Step Purification Breathing Technique
Sit in *Vairocana* and visualise your body as an empty, clear, luminous shell. Within lie the three channels - central blue, right red, and left white. The two side channels start at the nostrils, running parallel to the central channel. All three meet four fingers below the navel.

The **right** channel is solar energy, representing anger, and the bile humour - the fire element. The **left** channel is lunar, representing ignorance or delusion, and phlegm humour - the earth and water elements of the body. The **central** channel is wind energy representing desire or attachment. The imbalances of the right, left, and central channels are symbolised respectively by a snake, pig, and rooster. They in turn are considered the three fundamental poisons of conditioned human existence, the primary root cause of all worldly sufferings.

Maintain this visualisation of the body's pure dimension for a while, making sure that the thumb presses the root of the ring finger, making a partial *vajra* fist.

The purification breathing exercises should follow the following sequence:

## 1. Cleansing red energy (anger) from the right nostril
Starting with hands on lap, close your left nostril with the left index finger, and inhale while lifting the right index finger upwards from the lap towards the nose. Visualise drawing in pure five-coloured rainbow light through the right nostril, bringing it down the right channel, your right finger turning downwards, past the chest. When the finger reaches the point of the navel, turn your hand upwards, leading the energy up the left channel. When the right finger reaches the level of the left nostril, release the left finger from the left nostril, closing the right nostril with the right finger. Exhale all impurities of bile and anger, visualising this as a red smoke being expelled from the left nostril.

## 2. Cleansing white energy (ignorance) from the left nostril.

This time inhale through the left nostril, letting the left finger lead down the left channel then back up again. Slowly release the right finger from the right nostril when the left finger is brought up to the level of the left nostril. Close the left nostril with the left finger while exhaling, visualising the release of all ignorance, delusion and phlegm imbalances escaping from the nostril as a whitish, grey smoke.

## 3. Cleansing all channels

Next, inhale with both nostrils, guiding the energy downwards with both hands, before bringing them back to the nose. As you breathe in, visualise light entering and cleansing all the channels. When both hands reach the level of the nose, exhale and visualise yourself dispelling attachment, ego and all *rLung* imbalances as a dark smoke. Lower both hands to the original position.

These three breaths form a single cycle. The sequence is repeated three times to complete the nine breaths. This is followed by the practice of the vajra recitation with seven breaths; inhaling with white *Om*, holding with *red A*, and exhaling with *blue Hung*.

## Four Stages of Practice

Dream yoga has four stages of practice:

## 1. Body Position

The body should rest on the right side, left arm on the body; right little finger covering the right nostril.

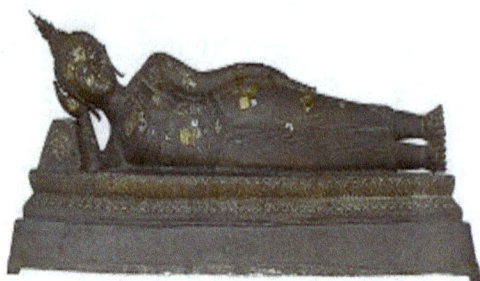

## 2. Time

Dream Yoga is practised at night, especially when the stars are shining, and energetically we are ready to sleep. At this time, our lunar energy starts to circulate in our channels, an ideal time for dream yoga. Therefore, energetically, sleeping during the day is unhealthy, except during a Dream Yoga retreat when it becomes part of the training.

## 3. Location

The seat of visualisation is the throat chakra, as it is the door of dreams. Starting here makes it easier to catch the dream. People who find it difficult to visualise the throat chakra may use either the head or heart chakra.

## 4. Visualisation

Use the figure below - the visualisation of *Om A Nu Ta Ra* (ༀ་ཨ་ནུ་ཏ་ར) with the syllable *Hung* in the centre - as a visualisation exercise in preparation to catch your dream.

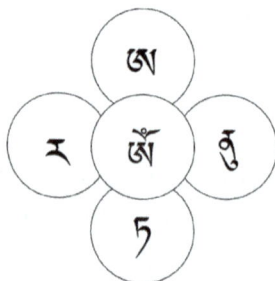

## The Four Processes in Dream Yoga

The actual visualisation sequence of Dream Yoga is called the **Four Processes**

| Catch |
| Purify |
| Overcome fear |
| Illusion |

### Process One: Catch (The Dream)

Starting the practice of dream yoga is like 'entering into the dream yoga house'. The entrance of the building is called 'Catching the dream', which means staying in a state of active, still awareness while dreaming. Several methods can be used to do this:

- Meditate on the empty body and channels
- Sleep with mindful, gentle breath
- Focus strongly on the desire of catching your dream
- Visualise a small white or red ball (*Thigle*)
- Visualise a syllable or letter
- Recite a mantra (e.g. *Om A Nu Ta Ra*) as much as possible until you sleep

### Mantra Visualisation

Meditate and visualise the mind as clear and pure. With the mantra recitation, visualise either a small, red ball of light at the throat or heart, or the whole body as red light.

A simpler method to catch the dream is to repeatedly imagine during the day that no matter what is experienced, all is merely a dream state. The more this is successfully practised, the greater the likelihood of becoming fully aware while dreaming. Practising this technique continuously develops ability in visualisation which is necessary to attaining success in dream yoga.

## Process Two: Purify

When the dream is caught, it must be purified with **Transformation**, **Multiplication**, and **Space Travelling**.

The **transformation** exercise helps to free the mind from logical thought, which is the main cause of conflicts and tensions, as for every emotion people invariably attempt to have a logical explanation, linked to cause and effect. The aim of this exercise is to make the impossible possible. Reality is a mental creation, as all existence is based on our thoughts and our beliefs. So if one's mind changes, then all shifts accordingly as the mind is a master creator of all.

- *Step one*: *Transformation of the Subject* – in dream state, self becomes transformed
- *Step two*: *Transformation of the Object* refers to changing an object perceived during a dream into another. At the beginning, it is easier to start with similar sized objects, such as changing a flower or cup into a bottle, before gradually increasing the sizes of the objects, such as changing a house into a mountain. Big objects may also be reduced in size. For example, transforming a table from a mustard seed into a house and back again to a mustard seed. Likewise, it is possible to play with colours - white to black, black to white, or whichever colour preferred.

**Multiplication.** Multiplying self is a technique in transforming dreams. If starting with oneself, it is easier to start with

low numbers such as 2x2 or 4x4, before multiplying the self exponentially to *ad infinitum*. If working on self is hard, start with objects first.
- Multiplying objects. Similarly begin with small objects before going on to medium size and large objects.

**Space Travelling,** the third dream purification technique, can be used to overcome the logical construct of distance and time. In the actual dream this is done by moving the self from within a room to outside a building, penetrating walls, or instantly transporting the self to any desired place, country or continent. Or even teleporting to a different dimension - the planets, stars and beyond, to the pure lands. If the dreamer succeeds in visiting the pure lands, visualise its different directions *Vajra* (east); *Ratna* (south), *Padma* (west), and the *Karma* (north). In the centre (straight up) is the *Buddha* dimension.

### Process three: Overcoming Fear
Once able to purify dreams, overcoming fear becomes the next obstacle, which can be dealt with through the three mental exercises of:
- *Illusory Meditation*: The dream practitioner meditates on the illusionary nature of the mind, to remind the self that all dreams entering our own mind do not have an existence outside of it. Therefore, like all our thoughts, all manifestations from our mind are mere illusions. That the pure nature of the mind is nothingness.
- *Interdependent Antidote*: The dream practitioner searches for the primary cause, going through primary and then secondary causes which led to the event itself, differentiating effect from cause.
- *Adverse Interdependence*: Based on a result or a consequence, the dreamer tracks back to the cause.

## Process Four: Dream is Illusion

When we realise, while dreaming, that our dream is merely a projection of our mind, and thus an illusion, we become aware of the true nature of the mind. Such awareness can also be perceived during waking state. In dreaming there is no separation between subject and object, which means there is no difference between mind and matter. All that manifests in the dream (colours, forms, odours, sound, touch, taste) is no different from the mind itself. The Tibetan term is *nangsem yerme* non-separation of appearance and mind. Therefore the dream is a total illusion.

## The Dream Yoga Retreat Practice

Going on a retreat allows for dream yoga practice day and night. However, careful preparations and **guidance from a qualified teacher** are required to make the retreat a success.

## Preparation
### Dream Yoga Day Practice
- Be mindful, perceive all action as a permanent dream state, whether meditating, eating, cleaning, or working.
- Meditate on the illusionary body, always keeping in mind that the body is illusory. From time to time, look into a mirror and talk to your image, as a perfect example of your illusionary body.
- From time to time chant the mantra.
- Do a breathing exercise: counting numbers or visualising colours.

| Breath | Inhale | Hold | Exhale |
|---|---|---|---|
| Count till | 4 | 4 | 4 |
| Or count till | 4 | 3 | 5 |
| Visualise | white | red | blue |

During the training, there should be balanced intervals of concentration and relaxation. Don't strain by over concentrating. It is very important to maintain a good balance between concentration and relaxation, much like playing a piano or driving a car. A driver pays just enough attention to avoid accidents, yet stays sufficiently relaxed, able to drive for many hours.

### Dream Yoga Night Practice

1. Meditate on an empty body and channels.
2. Visualise a red light at the throat, inside the central channel.
3. Chant the mantra: **Om A Nu Ta Ra**
4. Start by sleeping prone, and then slowly move into the Lion or Buddha position.
5. *Remind yourself "I am doing Dream Yoga: catching the dream".*
6. Focus on the red light, from time to time rest and focus on breathing.

*Stop meditation after 20 minutes*

## The Five Wisdoms ཡེ་ཤེས་ལྔ་ (*ye shes lnga*)

This section is about embryology in subtle anatomy. It explains how our spiritual practice is connected with the newly born baby, which in fact emerges with full realisation. After birth it depends on the individual whether this potential is achieved.

Usually, the prenatal period can be divided into 10 stages in which different *rLung* energies are supporting the child in later life.

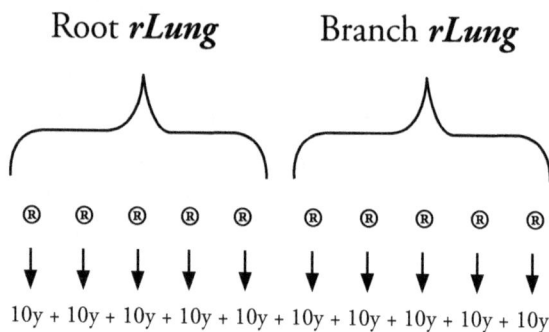

**Root *rLung***      **Branch *rLung***

Ⓡ   Ⓡ   Ⓡ   Ⓡ   Ⓡ    Ⓡ   Ⓡ   Ⓡ   Ⓡ   Ⓡ

↓   ↓   ↓   ↓   ↓    ↓   ↓   ↓   ↓   ↓

10y + 10y + 10y + 10y + 10y + 10y + 10y + 10y + 10y + 10y

During these stages the consciousness experiences various kinds of primordial awareness, called *ye shes lNga* (ཡེ་ཤེས་ལྔ་). Also known as the **Five Wisdoms of the Five Buddhas**, they denote the true nature of our mind. If we can accomplish these five wisdoms, we will reach realisation.

Therefore from the very beginning, the human body has within itself the seed for realisation. The table below explains how these five wisdoms are naturally inherent within us.

*sNgon Byang* (སྔོན་བྱང་།) means completely pure. Our mind consciousness from the beginning is completely pure.

The explanations of the five wisdoms are derived from the Tibetan Buddhist *Vajrayana* practice.

| ཡེ་ཤེས་ | Wisdom | Embryonic stage |
|---|---|---|
| *me long ye shes* | Mirror-like wisdom | Lunar energy which in subtle anatomy is also the father's energy. This energy is experienced when consciousness enters the sperm, a feeling like being a mirror. This is pure awareness and a full ability to reflect. During this period the mind can reflect all. Feelings of consciousness come from past life. |
| *nyam nyid ye shes* | Wisdom of equality | The wisdom of equality is solar energy, inside the female egg. At the moment of conception, when the sperm enters with consciousness into the egg, the consciousness is a feeling of total equanimity, a balance of male and female, hot and cold, solar and lunar. |
| *sor tog ye shes* | Discriminating wisdom or wisdom of individual awareness | When the foetus starts growing, consciousness experiences extreme orgasmic pleasure, lasting five weeks. This is *lhankyi gava* - substantial pleasure or bliss. The bliss which is born and connected with us - *sor tog ye shes*. |
| *cha drub ye shes* | Accomplishing wisdom | After these five weeks many different channels and chakras develop. Many disappear while others grow. rLung sem spreads and grows with pleasure. A few billion channels grow. During this time *cha drub ye shes* stays for many months. Even after birth, channels continue disappearing or growing. |
| *chö ying ye shes* | All pervading wisdom or dharma state wisdom | Baby is completely formed and all channels, hair, skin and internal organs are developed. *chö ying ye shes* is present. |

Most *Buddhas* are pictured seated on a lotus flower. The sun and moon symbols contained within represent the first two wisdoms portraying the beginning of life, the lotus flower itself representing purity. The child is like a lotus flower growing from dirty mud, able to stay pure even if its mother eats impure food and provides tainted energy to the baby. All men and women are born like lotus flowers, containing both solar and lunar energy. The two wisdoms of *me long ye shes* and *nyam nyid ye shes* lie within this purity.

## Creation Practice

### The Power of Medicine Buddha Visualisation

Visualise a lotus flower, and on it a moon and a sun disc. In the centre of the flower is the syllable *Hung* - the symbol of the third wisdom, *sor tog ye shes*.

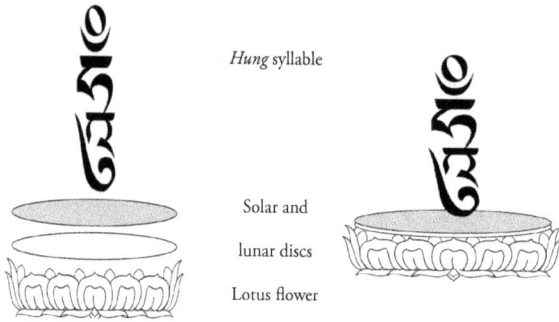

*Hung* syllable

Solar and

lunar discs

Lotus flower

Focus on the syllable, say *hung* and visualise your transformation into the *Medicine Buddha*. Your body has changed - each part totally perfect, your whole body a deep sky blue; your sense organs perfectly attuned, your hair, all parts of your body including energy and channels growing in you, is complete perfection. This is the wisdom of accomplishment, *cha drub ye shes* the perfection of *Medicine Buddha*.

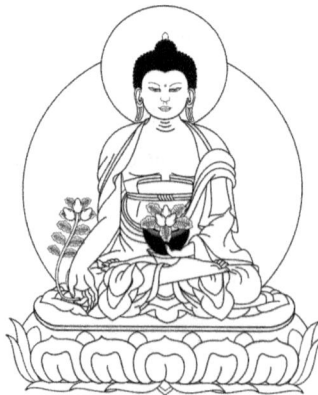

Begin the purification practice, focusing your mind and visualising yourself as *Medicine Buddha*. Recite the Medicine Buddha mantra and visualise light emerging from your heart and radiating into all directions to purify the universe. This is *chö ying ye shes*, the wisdom of the *dharma* state.

## Transform yourself into Medicine Buddha

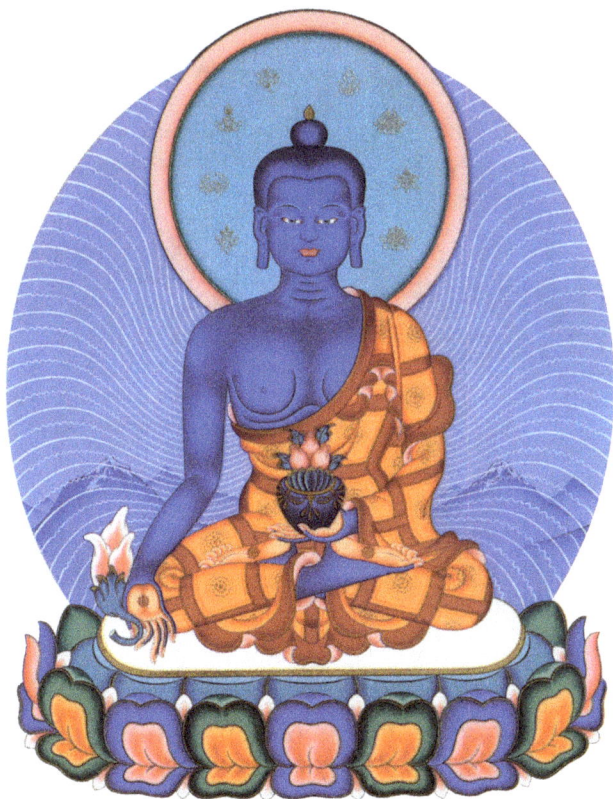

Space

Lotus

Moon *me long ye shes*

Sun *nyam nyid ye shes*

Seed syllable *sor tog ye shes*

Buddha *cha drub ye shes*

Radiation *chö ying ye shes*

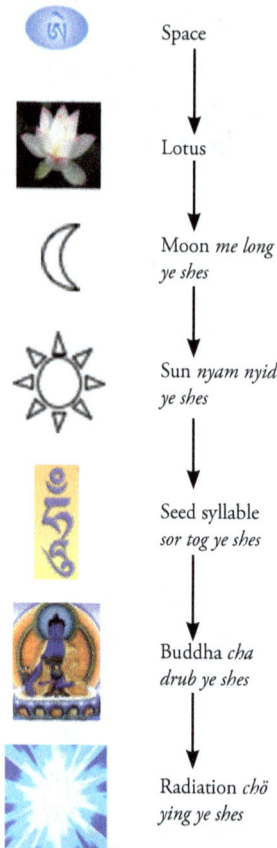

*Medicine Buddha* visualisation practice embraces a psychological idea: bad childhood experiences can cause blockages which we can remove by going back and replacing ourselves as a light body. This way the body returns to its original light form. This method is also used during visualisation practice in Tibetan Buddhism.

The second reason in visualising ourselves as *Medicine Buddha* is to develop and use this energy to benefit others. Becoming aware of this *Buddha*-like quality will help in reaching spiritual realisation. The basic idea is: *nothing is external, everything is internal.* In subtle anatomy there are different approaches to reach realisation. But first one must achieve a state of equilibrium, starting with a normal, stable mind. Confused minds lead to various forms of depression. It is only when the mind is calm and stable will it be possible to commence a practice towards spiritual realisation.

## Simple *Medicine Buddha* Meditation Practice

### *Step one*

Begin by focusing on a small object - a stone or plant - before moving on to a *Medicine Buddha* image. Or just concentrate on your breathing. Be mindful of the breath.

**Step two**
Visualise yourself as *Medicine Buddha*, chanting the mantra of *Hung* or *Hum*. Clearly see each part of your body as full of light; a union of emptiness and appearance.

**Step three**
At the centre of the heart chakra is a *Hung* syllable, surrounded by the *Medicine Buddha* mantra. It starts to radiate light. This light is offered to all Buddhas and enlightened beings, before going out to heal the entire universe, dissolving bad karma and providing the energy to all sentient beings. With the light you can heal, liberate, pacify, increase wisdom, gain positive spiritual power, energy, and so on.

**Step four**
Chant the Medicine Buddha mantra:

**TAYATHA OM BEKAZE BEKAZE MAHA BEKAZE**
**RAZA SAMUNG GATE SOHA**

While reciting the mantra, from time to time focus your mind on your body or a part of it. Concentrate your mind on the light. Think of the meaning of what you are chanting.

**Step five**
Everything dissolves into emptiness; then again everything illusory manifests as normal.

**Step six**
Make a dedication (compassionate thought) together with the mantra.

The visualisation and chanting of the *Medicine Buddha* practice described here is an important foundation to the development of dream yoga as a spiritual practice. Being able to strongly perform the mental visualisation required here leads to success in dream yoga practice.

# Conclusion

I hope this book offers readers a deeper understanding of the profound knowledge and rich history that ancient Tibetan medicine possesses on the importance of dream analysis. By introducing Buddhist cosmology and what we consider to make up the constitution of individuals, together with other key factors such as the environment, the seasons, and a person's state of mind, I have sought to explain the mysterious world of dreams.

As a medical practitioner, analysing dreams is an essential diagnostic tool that I use with my patients, one which has time and again proven to be invaluable in helping to diagnose disorders and prescribing effective treatments. However, the layman will also find the concepts and methods of dream analysis, together with examples of case studies that I have selected, useful in trying to understand how dreams may relate to events experienced in daily life.

For those who are keen and want to learn more about becoming a dream yoga practitioner, the journey will demand wholehearted dedication and serious, continuous daily practice. But the rewards are many.

And for the very few prepared to go all the way, they will tread the paths of the ancient dream yoga masters, aiming for the ultimate goal of blissful realisation, a rare achievement attained by only a few of even the Masters themselves.

But the main purpose of this book is to bring this ancient art of dream interpretation to the many. My hope is that this book will benefit them.

July 2013

Part 3

# Meaning of Dreams
## Typology, Glossary and Case Studies

# Dreams according to Typology

As a summary guide, the following table shows how dreams can be classified according to a person's typology - whether the dreamer is a *rLung, mKhris pa* or *Bad kan* person. The typology analysis is based on the colour, actions and feelings experienced during a dream and also by noting the dream setting and the time of sleep.

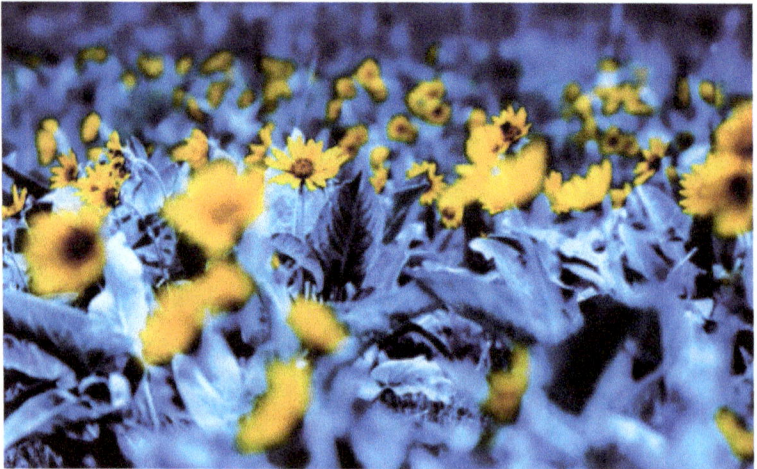

| | *rLung* | MKhris pa | *Bad kan* |
|---|---|---|---|
| **Colour** | Predominately blue, e.g. blue flowers, dress in blue, blue houses; also sky blue, dark blue and black (especially black animals). | Dreams are yellow and red, e.g. red and yellow flowers, herbs, clothes and houses. | Dreams are white: white clothes, flowers, and objects such as snow, white houses, buildings etc. |
| **Actions and emotions** | Often includes climbing a mountain or stairs, being in a plane or flying.<br><br>Generally associated with very light, unstable, changing feelings. You may be talking to people when the scene suddenly changes and you find yourself walking elsewhere, again suddenly changing to the middle of a city.<br><br>Emotions in *rLung* dreams are unsettled, nervous and desirous e.g wishing for good food, money, material objects. | Generally, strong and clear dreams. Warm or heat sensations e.g. shining sun, or burning fire.<br><br>The emotional tone generally includes anger/ pride, e.g. *mKhris pa* people get angry with others or feel that their pride has been affected because someone has done something to them. | Stable and strong dreams with feelings of cool or cold.<br><br>In *Bad kan* dreams a person may be speaking calmly for a long time. Themes are of a stable lifestyle.<br><br>Feelings are good with positive sensations; *Bad kan* people are very patient. |
| **Environment** | The dreams are situated in forests with wind element being present. | In a natural environment the sun may be shining, there may be a lightening flash, bright lights, shouting, stars and fires. Dreams may be affected by a hot environment, e.g. sleeping near a candle, lighter or open fire may create dreams of lying in the sun, near strong heat, or a burning fire. | In a dream where the person is in a natural environment there will be birds, clouds, mountains, rivers, oceans and lakes. |
| **Time** | Early morning, evening and the summer season. | Midnight, late afternoon or autumn season. | Late evening, early morning, spring and early summer seasons. |

127

# Some Dream Case Studies

The following are actual studies of dreams which I analysed for some of my students during dream workshops or with patients. A few I have taken from my own dreams. The ones here have been chosen as they show clearly the connection between dreams and our daily life.

## Ants (Difficulties)

*One day I had what seemed to be a fairly normal dream. I was conducting a course in Rome, and surrounded by many people. Then suddenly when I was trying to go somewhere, my path was impeded by an army of small ants, making it difficult to reach where I was trying to go. Eventually, I arrived at my destination - another city with many people and large buildings. The dream was rather long but when I woke up I had a clear memory of the ants.*

*Ants are a symbol of having difficulties with others so I thought I might have a problem with someone that day and carefully tried to avoid any potential conflict. But at the end of that day I still was unable to avoid difficulty with a particular person. The symbol in this reflective dream was the ants, which was only a small part of a long dream, and the situation which I faced was also a simple problem that was later easily rectified. The point here is that to focus on a symbol and emphasise its importance would have made the small problem unnecessarily larger than it was.*

## Fire (Bile Imbalance)

*One night I dreamt that I was making a fire with pieces of wood and I felt really hot. When I woke up I thought the dream might be symbolising something positive as fire and wood dreams are usually good.*

*After two or three hours I started to feel slightly off colour and developed a headache. Slowly the headache became stronger and as I became feverish, I remembered my dream; I perceived that my bile energies might be unbalanced so I washed my head with really cold water and began to feel much better. The connection between my energy levels (mkris pa) and the dream were clear and accurate.*

## Fish (Fertility)

Fish is a common dream symbol. The examples here give an insight in how they might surface in various dreams.

*A university friend once told me about a dream where he was fishing and caught a fish, and asked me what this meant. I replied that perhaps somebody connected with him would become pregnant, a friend or his own girlfriend, the latter to which he replied as being impossible. A month later he told me his girlfriend was pregnant.*

*This is just one example, I have verified the fish symbol in dreams with many people and I have seen that when a person dreams of fishing and catching fish it is a precise symbol of birth or rebirth.*

*Another person told me once that he dreamt about dead fish that were rotten and giving off a very strong smell. This man had health problems and his dream was directly connected to his state of health.*

Animals like fish, snakes and other reptiles are all considered to be fish symbols when they appear in water. They are all very flexible in movement and when they move well within dreams, it is a symbol of circulating energy.

*In Italy a lady asked about a recurring dream whereby she enters the deep part of the ocean and swims like a fish seeing many species of aquatic animals around her. I thought that it was possibly a karmic dream where she might have been a fish in a past life. I did not explain this to her as it might have upset her, it being highly possible to have dreams of previous existences.*

### Rats (Fortune)
*A person once asked me about a very clear dream he had in which he saw a white rat in his room being chased by a cat. He was pleased as he succeeded in stopping the cat from catching the rat. In the dream the cat and the rat seemed very real.*

*I explained that the rat was a sign of good fortune and money. A few weeks later he told me he won a considerable amount of money gambling.*

I read another text about dreams which says that if a person dreams that the cat actually catches the rat it is an indication of extreme good fortune.

In Tibetan Buddhism there are Tantric rituals that bring good fortune and if after attending the ritual or puja the participants see a dead mouse or rat that day or the next day they are assured of good fortune.

In Buddhist art there are many Deities of good fortune such as *Zhambala* and *Namsya* and in their hand is an animal that look much like a rat and these animals appear to be vomiting jewels. Perhaps then we shouldn't kill mice in our homes but rather keep them for good fortune!

## Blindness (Liver)

*A patient of mine despite very good eyesight repeatedly had a strange dream in which she could not see very much at all, everything appearing hazy. After some time her sight deteriorated to the point where her vision became blurred. My diagnosis was rLung disorder in the liver and I gave her medicine for the condition. Gradually her sight cleared and she began to see more clearly in her dreams.*

*Another patient had a liver problem due to alcohol. In Tibetan medicine this condition is treated with the season taken into account as the elements increase and decrease according to seasonal time of the year. Therefore during the season when the liver function was high this patient would encounter blindness in his dreams. In them, there would be no light or he often dreamt that it was night time or he was trying to do something in the dark. Even when he dreamt it was day, he still would not be able to see clearly.*

This is typical because during the time when the liver function increased, his dreams would be dark and during the season when the liver function decreased, his dreams would clear. This shows how the change in season and the elements influence the function of our organs and affect the pattern of our dreams.

## Moon (Death of a Master)

*In Lhasa once, I dreamt it was night and there was a very bright full moon. As I thought "Oh, what a beautiful moon", a black cloud suddenly covered the moon and everything be-*

131

*came dark. I woke up and wondered why I had this very nega-*
*tive dream; that perhaps something was wrong with one of my*
*Teachers. When I returned home six months later, I was told*
*that a very famous Terton Master (alag Tergan) passed away*
*during the time of my dream.*

## Prophetic dream

*A girl had a dream in which she had sex with a man and felt*
*good about it. In the middle of the sexual act, she woke and*
*found it was morning. Being a virgin it was also the first time*
*she had the sensation of sex. A few weeks later, the man in her*
*dream also dreamt he had sex with her. His dream happened as*
*well early in the morning. That day they unexpectedly met and*
*had sex together.*

## Snakes (Money and Conflict)

*A lady asked me about a dream in which a person gave her a*
*lamp to hold. Within the lamp, she saw many animals, includ-*
*ing fish and snakes. I know this to be a very good symbol for re-*
*ceiving a lot of money. She thought it could possibly mean that*
*she herself had neither much money, nor the means to make it.*
*After a couple of months she returned very happy to tell me that*
*the dream symbol was accurate and that she had come into a*
*considerable amount of money.*

The snake symbol in dreams is also quite precise in identify-
ing emotional conflicts. When patients tell me about their
dreams of snakes, my analysis usually reveals deep-seated
conflicts with other people.

*A friend of mine often dreams about snakes. At first, I thought*
*that his dreams were connected with Nagas, a particular type*
*of nocturnal disturbance. Later I discovered his snake dreams*

*were mainly related to the serious problems he was facing with his girlfriend and the strong resentment they harboured against each other. In fact they really hated each other to the point where the girlfriend said that she wanted to kill him.*

*I asked him how the snakes moved in his dreams and he said that he would be walking along and he would think that there might be snakes around, whereupon he would immediately become tense. As soon as he thought that, snakes would then appear and he would become very frightened, even though they might not attack him.*

*Other times in his dreams he would be holding a bag full of snakes and be rooted to the spot, unable to move or run away. In these dreams he would always be fearful, feeling himself surrounded by snakes either trying to attack him or remaining passive.*

*I asked if he was scared of his girlfriend and he answered yes! So I enquired why he is afraid of his girlfriend, to describe the feeling and if it was the same feeling he had in his dreams. He said that it was difficult for him to feel deeply in love with her as there was always the strange underlying feeling of fear similar to what he experienced in his dreams. I informed him that the snake in his dream was actually the manifestation of his girlfriend's anger and hate towards him.*

*I told him to try and improve his relationship with his girlfriend, to be especially nice to her and helping her to relax. Somehow he succeeded in doing that and when his girlfriend became happy again, her anger subsided altogether, and his dreams of snakes gradually decreased. But now and then, when his girlfriend gets angry with him, his dreams of snakes would return, accompanied by the very same frightened feelings he used to have.*

## Falling Teeth (Death)

*I had a dream that my lower teeth were falling out. The dream started about seven in the morning and as my teeth started to fall out I tried to push them back into my gum with my tongue, one tooth still managing to fall out totally. The dream was so vivid that I woke up thinking I lost a tooth, but happily found all my teeth still intact when I checked.*

*A month or so later, I dreamt the same thing vividly again. This time, I thought that perhaps something bad had happened to a relative on my mother's side as both dreams were about my lower teeth. Six or eight months later my uncle on my mother's side passed away. I remained concerned as I had the same dream twice. A month later another relative on my mother's side passed away again.*

## Wrong Sleeping Position

*A friend of mine, a Buddhist monk, had almost nightly bad dreams. He dreamt of death symbols and being in dangerous situations. I knew this monk quite well, and that he was a very good practitioner, so I wondered why he would have these dreams. I asked him to show me his sleeping position. He lay on his back and crossed his ankles. I asked him to change his position to sleeping on his right side. His negative dreams ceased when he did so.*

# Glossary of Dream Symbols

This comprehensive list of dream symbols is an invaluable guide to gauge the different meanings behind the rich variety of objects appearing within a person's dream. It provides an instant reference, especially to a novice dream practitioner seeking to decipher the positive or negative meanings behind dream symbols.

| Symbol | Expression in Dream | Meaning |
|--------|---------------------|---------|
| Action | Acting out of control | Negative symbol, negative meaning |
| Age | Feeling old age or becoming sick | Negative symbol, negative meaning |
| Animals | Strange looking animals | Positive symbol, positive meaning |
| Animals | Attacking dogs, wolves, monkeys, tigers, foxes or other such angry animals | Symbolises illness or its onset. Negative symbol, negative meaning |
| Babies | Babies and children with dark skin and poor complexion | Negative health indicator. Negative symbol, negative meaning |
| Babies | Babies and children with bright skin and good complexion | Positive symbol, positive meaning |
| Birds | Strange looking birds | Positive symbol, positive meaning |
| Birth | Giving birth to a baby with good skin and complexion | Positive symbol, positive meaning |
| Biting | Animal bites, bleeding wounds | Solving a problem. Negative symbol with positive meaning |
| Biting | Animal bites but no bleeding wounds | Indicates becoming seriously ill. Negative symbol, negative meaning |
| Blood | Menstruation | Sign of elimination. Positive symbol, positive meaning |
| Blood | Bloody or bleeding body (any part) | Negative symbol with positive meaning |
| Boat | Travelling by boat | Positive symbol, positive meaning |
| Bridge | Broken bridges or rivers without bridges | Negative symbol, negative meaning |
| Buddha | Buddha, Deities, Gods of any religions | Positive symbol, positive meaning |

| Buildings | Climbing up a clean or new building | Happiness. Positive symbol, positive meaning |
| Buildings | Falling down a building | Negative symbol, negative meaning |
| Buildings | Constructing buildings and roads | Positive symbol, positive meaning |
| Buildings | Appearing in the dream | Negative symbol with positive meaning |
| Cats | Cats that are not your own, strange looking cats seeking something | Indicates presence of disturbed beings. Positive symbol with negative meaning |
| Celebrities | Celebrities, famous movie stars | Positive symbol, positive meaning |
| Cemetery | Dead bodies or strong negative energies attacking, sucking energy, weakening you | Manifestation of a dead person. Negative symbol, negative meaning |
| Children | Vital young children between the ages of eight and twelve especially dressed in yellow | Increase of energy and good fortune. Positive symbol, positive meaning |
| Children | Vital young children between eight and twelve dressed in white | Represent peace, absence of illness. Positive symbol, positive meaning |
| Circles | Paintings with squares and circles | Positive symbol, positive meaning |
| City | Good clean places such as towns, cities and villages | Positive symbol, positive meaning |
| Cleaning | Cleaning house and throwing out rubbish | Indicates financial problems. Positive symbol with negative meaning |
| Clothes | Finding good clothes with embroidery or decorations | Fame. Positive symbol, positive meaning |
| Clothes | Washing | Positive symbol, positive meaning |
| Clothes | Ugly or poor clothing | Negative symbol, negative meaning |
| Containers | Full containers in the kitchen | Positive symbol, positive meaning |
| Containers | Empty containers | Negative symbol, negative meaning |
| Cows | Riding cows, horses or other kinds of animals (not in a southerly direction) | Positive symbol, positive meaning |
| Crystal | Clear, clean glass, crystal or mirrors | Positive symbol, positive meaning |
| Dalai Lama | Or other holy people, teachers | Positive symbol, positive meaning |
| Darkness | Darkness falling, or night time | Negative symbol, negative meaning |
| Death | Dreaming that you are dead | Negative symbol with positive meaning |
| Death | In tantric teachings, seeing, touching or carrying dead bodies | Represent *siddhis*. Negative symbol with positive meaning |

| | | |
|---|---|---|
| Deceased | Dead persons inviting you to eat, drink, dance and go elsewhere | Means losing energy and dying. Positive symbol with negative meaning |
| Diarrhoea | If a person is doing a purification practice such as *Vajrasattva* | Symbolises purification, negative energies leaving the body. Negative symbol with positive meaning |
| Dirt | Having a very dirty body or being in a dirty environment | Negative symbol, negative meaning |
| Dirty place | Leaving a dirty place | Positive symbol, positive meaning |
| Disease | Feeling old or becoming sick | Negative symbol, negative meaning |
| Dogs | Strange looking dogs, not your own pets | Presence of disturbed beings. Positive symbol with negative meaning |
| Door | Moving away from a door | Negative symbol, negative meaning |
| Downwards Direction | Travelling in any downward direction | Negative symbol, negative meaning |
| Drink | Eating dirty food and drinking dirty water or tea | Symbolise illness. Negative symbol, negative meaning |
| Drink | Drinking black tea, oil or brown liquids | Positive symbol with negative meaning |
| East | Any appearance | Positive symbol, positive meaning |
| Eclipse | Appearing anywhere | Means death of a great Master. Negative symbol, negative meaning |
| Excretion | As part of the birth process or releasing stool | Sign of elimination. Positive symbol, positive meaning |
| Faeces | Appearing anywhere, body covered in faeces | Symbol of fortune and wealth. Negative symbol with positive meaning |
| Fight | Winning against another person | Positive symbol, positive meaning |
| Fire | Fire around the body | Positive symbol, positive meaning |
| Fire | Appearing anywhere | Negative symbol with positive meaning |
| Fish | Dead fish | Energy blockage, work or activities may meet problems. Negative symbol, negative meaning |
| Fish | Especially golden or yellow fish | Symbol of increasing fortune, power or energy. Positive symbol, positive meaning |
| Fish | Fish eating a person | Symbol of life coming to an end. Positive symbol with negative meaning |

| | | |
|---|---|---|
| Fish | Female dreaming about catching a fish | Indicates pregnancy – self, family member, or friend. Positive symbol, positive meaning |
| Flags | Dreaming of your own flag | Symbol of success. Positive symbol, positive meaning |
| Flags | Weapons or flags inside your home | Indicates an external opposing energy arriving to disturb. Positive symbol with negative meaning |
| Flies | Any appearance | Negative symbol, negative meaning |
| Flying | Flying by airplanes or in the sky | Positive symbol, positive meaning |
| Flood | Floods washing all away | Negative symbol with positive meaning |
| Flood | Storms and floods with dirty water | Negative symbol, negative meaning |
| Flowers | Any kind, especially white flowers | Positive symbol, positive meaning |
| Flowers | Planting flowers, fresh, cut flowers | Symbol of fresh energy and new beginning. Positive symbol, positive meaning |
| Food | Eating plenty of healthy, delicious food | Positive symbol, positive meaning |
| Food | Begging for money or food | Negative symbol, negative meaning |
| Food | Eating dirty food or drinking dirty water/tea | Symbolises illness. Negative symbol, negative meaning |
| Forests | Appearing in any form | Positive symbol, positive meaning |
| Frogs | Frogs in river or lake with other water creatures | Symbolises diseases e.g. lymphatic and joint problems. Positive symbol with negative meaning |
| Fruits | Trees with ripe fruit | Positive symbol, positive meaning |
| Garbage | Dirty places with garbage | Negative symbol, negative meaning |
| Gems | Such as coral or turquoise | Positive symbol, positive meaning |
| Gold | Especially gold powder | Represents death, difficulties in succeeding in a mission. Positive symbol with negative meaning |
| Gold | Appearing to a Buddhist practitioner | Shows improving practice. Positive symbol, positive meaning |
| Ground | A person falling down and standing again | Positive symbol, positive meaning |
| Grubs | Appearance of any kind | Negative symbol, negative meaning |
| Hair | Cutting your hair or shaving | Knowledge or natural power is decreasing. Negative symbol, negative meaning |

| | | |
|---|---|---|
| Hair | Own hair is growing | Knowledge or natural power is increasing. Positive symbol, positive meaning |
| Hats | Good hats | Indicates high position in office. Positive symbol, positive meaning |
| Hats | Losing your hat or shoes | Negative symbol, negative meaning |
| Herbs | Finding or collecting herbs | Positive symbol, positive meaning |
| Herbs | Dried herbs | Negative symbol, negative meaning |
| Holidays | Going on holidays | Indicates sadness or problems with the mind. Positive symbol with negative meaning |
| Horses | Riding cows, horses or other kinds of animals (not in southerly direction) | Positive symbol, positive meaning |
| House | Broken houses | Negative symbol, negative meaning |
| House | Difficulty in getting out of a house | Negative symbol, negative meaning |
| Insects | Insects like cockroaches crawling on your body | Symbolising illness. Negative symbol, negative meaning |
| Kitchen | Full containers in the kitchen | Positive symbol, positive meaning |
| Lake | Crossing a river or a lake without any problems | Sign of positive endeavour bringing success at work. Positive symbol, positive meaning |
| Lake | Entering a dirty river or lake | Negative symbol, negative meaning |
| Loneliness | Travelling alone, feeling lonely, or without friends | Warnings of obstacles in life and karmic hindrances. Negative symbol, negative meaning |
| Magic | Magic powers used on self | Negative symbol, negative meaning |
| Menstruation | Having menstruation | Sign of elimination, Positive symbol, positive meaning |
| Meat | Eating raw meat | Indicates problems. Positive symbol with negative meaning |
| Meat | For *Chod* practitioners eating fresh, raw meat full of blood | Symbolises good practice. Positive symbol, positive meaning |
| Mirror | Clear, clean glass, crystal or mirrors | Positive symbol, positive meaning |
| Mirror | Looking in the mirror | Indicates obstacles. Positive symbol with negative meaning |
| Money | Begging for money or food | Negative symbol, negative meaning |
| Moon | In Tibetan culture | Represents Masters and Teachers. Positive symbol, positive meaning |

139

| Moon | Moon covered by clouds and there is no light | Symbolises death of a teacher or master. Negative symbol, negative meaning |
|------|------|------|
| Mountain | Climbing or reaching the top of a mountain | Happiness. Positive symbol, positive meaning |
| Mountain | Walking or falling down a mountain, down large rocks or travelling in any downward direction | Negative symbol, negative meaning |
| Mounts | Riding horses or donkeys without a saddle while naked | Means no success in work or daily activities. Negative symbol, negative meaning |
| Mounts | Donkeys, camels and horses | Animals symbolise the southerly direction and death. Negative symbol, negative meaning |
| Music | Appearing in any form | Symbol relates to fame. Positive symbol, positive meaning |
| Night | Falling darkness, dreaming that it is night time | Negative symbol, negative meaning |
| North | Appearing in any form | Positive symbol, positive meaning |
| Offerings | Making offerings | Positive symbol, positive meaning |
| Painting | Paintings with squares and circles | Positive symbol, positive meaning |
| Parents | Respect from your parents | Positive symbol, positive meaning |
| Place | Strange places, never visited before especially if you are alone in the dream | Means leaving for your next life. Positive symbol with negative meaning |
| Poison | Poisonous herbs and flowers | Negative symbol with positive meaning |
| Losing Possession | Losing your weapons or your possessions | Negative symbol, negative meaning |
| Rain | Heavy rains | Negative symbol with positive meaning |
| Rats and mice | Appearing anywhere | Symbol of good fortune. Positive symbol, positive meaning |
| Red | E.g. red flowers or red dress | Controlling function, represents death. Positive symbol with negative meaning |
| River | Crossing a river without any problems | Sign of positive endeavour and success at work. Positive symbol, positive meaning |
| River | Entering a dirty river or lake | Negative symbol, negative meaning |
| River | Broken bridges or rivers without bridges | Negative symbol, negative meaning |

| | | |
|---|---|---|
| Roads | Constructing buildings and roads | Positive symbol, positive meaning |
| Roads | Bumpy, narrow roads | Meaning your positive energy is diminishing. Negative symbol, negative meaning |
| Sex | Experiencing nice sensations without loss of sperm | Special transmission from *Dakas* or *Dakinis*. Positive symbol, positive meaning |
| Sex | Male dreaming about sex with ejaculation | Your energy taken by negative female energy. Positive symbol with negative meaning |
| Sex | Female dreaming about sex and getting pregnant | Disturbing negative energy. Positive symbol with negative meaning |
| Ship | Travelling by boat or ship | Positive symbol, positive meaning |
| Shoes | Good, clean or new shoes | Success in life and work. Positive symbol, positive meaning |
| Shoes | Losing shoes | Negative symbol, negative meaning |
| Singing | Anywhere in the dream | Fame symbol. Positive symbol, positive meaning |
| Snakes | Snakes attacking or biting | Indicates joint or skin disease. Negative symbol, negative meaning |
| Snakes | White or silver snakes | Male energy is increasing, symbol is linked with *kundalini*. Negative symbol with positive meaning |
| Snakes | Yellow snakes, many intertwined like a knot | Strong symbol of money and great fortune. Negative symbol with positive meaning |
| Snow | Male dreaming about snow | Sign of good fortune. Positive symbol, positive meaning |
| Snow | Sick person dreaming about snow | Means overcoming illness. Positive symbol, positive meaning |
| Snow | Female dreaming about snow | Means problems will be resolved, confusions clarified, mental suffering ended. Positive symbol, positive meaning |
| Snow | Snow with wind | Negative symbol, negative meaning |
| South | In tantric teachings e.g. Yamantaka the south direction | Means Yama, Lord of Death. Negative symbol, negative meaning |
| Squares | Paintings with squares and circles | Positive symbol, positive meaning |
| Stairs | Climbing up stairs | Happiness. Positive symbol, positive meaning |
| Stairs | Going down stairs | Negative symbol, negative meaning |

| | | |
|---|---|---|
| Storm | Storms with gales that destroy | Negative symbol with positive meaning |
| Storm | Storms and floods with dirty water | Negative symbol, negative meaning |
| Sun | In Tibetan culture | Represents Masters and Teachers. Positive symbol, positive meaning |
| Sun | Anywhere in dream | Sign of happiness. Positive symbol, positive meaning |
| Sun | Covered by clouds and no light | Negative symbol, negative meaning |
| Sunrise | Rising sun at dawn | Symbolises arrival of light and happiness. Positive symbol, positive meaning |
| Tears | Crying in a dream with real tears | Negative symbol with positive meaning |
| Teeth | Upper teeth falling out | Death on father's side of the family. Negative symbol, negative meaning |
| Teeth | Lower teeth falling out | Indicates a death on the mother's side. Negative symbol, negative meaning |
| Tent | Broken tents | Negative symbol, negative meaning |
| Tent | Difficulty in getting out of a tent | Negative symbol, negative meaning |
| Town | Good clean towns, cities and villages | Positive symbol, positive meaning |
| Tree | Climbing up a tree | Happiness. Positive symbol, positive meaning |
| Tree | Any type of tree | Symbols of fresh energy and new beginning. Positive symbol, positive meaning |
| Tree | Dried trees | Negative symbol, negative meaning |
| Umbrellas | Anywhere | Indicates long life. Positive symbol, positive meaning |
| Upward direction | Walking uphill, looking up | Indicates successful practice. Positive symbol, positive meaning |
| Urine | Urinating | Sign of elimination. Positive symbol, positive meaning |
| Vajra | Receiving golden Vajra | For Buddhist practitioner symbolises good, spiritual practice and power. Positive symbol, positive meaning |
| Vomiting | If undergoing purification practices such as *Vajrasattva* | Symbolises purification. Negative symbol with positive meaning |

| Water | Dirty water | Indicates blocked channels, mental or physical problem (especially urination tract problems). Negative symbol, negative meaning |
|---|---|---|
| Water | Swimming in water, taking a shower | Purification dream. Positive symbols with positive meaning |
| Weapons | Weapons or flags inside the home | Indicates arrival of disturbing, external, opposing energy. Positive symbol with negative meaning |
| Weapons | Well-kept weapons such as guns or knifes | Symbols of protection. Positive symbol, positive meaning |
| Weapons | Losing one's weapons or possessions | Negative symbol, negative meaning |
| Wedding | Wedding party | Sign of death. Positive symbol with negative meaning |
| Weight | Losing weight | Negative symbol, negative meaning |
| West | In tantric teachings e.g. Yamantaka west direction | Indicates *Yama*, Lord of Death. Negative symbol, negative meaning |
| White | General appearance of white colour | Positive symbol, positive meaning |
| Wind | Gale force winds | Negative symbol with positive meaning |
| Wind | Snow with wind | Negative symbol, negative meaning |
| Window | Difficulty in getting out of a window | Negative symbol, negative meaning |

# Bibliography

Yuthok Yonten Gonpo. གསོ་རིག་རྒྱུད་བཞི། gso rig rgyud bzhi, THE FOUR MEDICAL TANTRAS, Tibet People's Publishing House, Lhasa.5th may.2006

Yuthok Yonten Gonpo, གཡུ་ཐོག་སྙིང་ཐིག gYuthok nying thig, Yuthok's heart teachings. National Publishing house Beijing. 2005

Lama Longdol. sklong rdol blama ngag dbang blo bzang, rmi lts sna tshogs dpyad thabs. THE DREAM INTERPRETATION. Gansu National Publisher. August 2002

Karmapa rangbyung rdoje, zabmo nangdon THE INNER TRUE MEANING, National Publisher. 2006

Sakyepa gyentsen pelsang. rdo rje lus kyi sbas bshad, THE VAJRA BODY EXPLANATION. National Publisher. 1991.

# Index

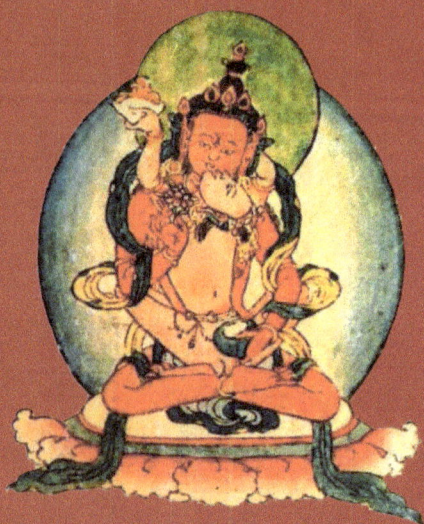

*Visualisation of
the Throat Chakra*

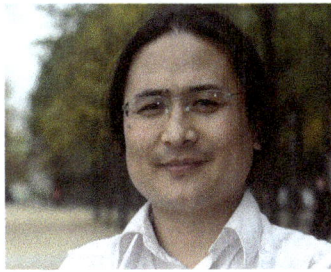

Dr. Nida Chenagtsang, a Tibetan doctor, Director of the International Academy for Traditional Tibetan Medicine (IATTM), is trained in modern and Traditional Tibetan Medicine and seen his writings translated into nine languages, including the sacred practice of Dream Yoga.

He is dedicated to training students globally in a comprehensive four year Tibetan Medicine programme, as well as in other modalities such as Ku Nye External Therapies, Dreams, Mantra Healing and Nejang Yoga, travelling tirelessly throughout Asia, Europe and the Americas to help set up over 20 International Academies for Traditional Tibetan Medicine (IATTM).

He has published many articles and books on ancient Tibetan Medicine, establishing important research areas and bringing back into current usage long forgotten traditional therapies. A founder of the Ngakmang Institute, he has also helped preserve and disseminate the Ngakpa culture in modern Tibetan society today.

Dr Tam Nguyen was born in Heidelberg, Germany, to Vietnamese parents, and grew up with both Asian and buddhist influences. She studied medicine at the University of Heidelberg, and is currently working in a hospital in Winterthur, Swirzerland. Since 2009 she has been studying Tibetan medicine with IATTM, and is currently both Executive Director and one of the teachers of IATTM.

www.ingramcontent.com/pod-product-compliance
Lightning Source LLC
LaVergne TN
LVHW021119080426
835510LV00012B/1760